Obstetrics
for the
House Officer

Second Edition

GW01066251

Obstetrics for the House Officer

Second Edition

William F. Rayburn, M.D.

Professor and Director
Division of Maternal-Fetal Medicine
Department of Obstetrics and Gynecology
University of Nebraska College of Medicine
Omaha, Nebraska

Justin P. Lavin, Jr., M.D.

Chief, Division of Obstetrics
Akron City Hospital
Professor
Department of Obstetrics and Gynecology
Northeastern Ohio Universities College of Medicine
Akron, Ohio

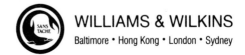

WILLIAMS & WILKINS

Baltimore • Hong Kong • London • Sydney

Editor: Nancy Collins
Associate Editor: Carol Eckhart
Copy Editor: Anne Schwartz
Design: JoAnne Janowiak
Illustration Planning: Wayne Hubbel
Production: Raymond E. Reter
Cover Design: Dan Psfisterer

Copyright (c) 1988
Williams & Wilkins
428 East Preston Street
Baltimore, MD 21202, USA

Accurate indications, adverse reactions, and dosage schedules for drugs are provided in this book, but it is possible that they may change. The reader is urged to review the package information data of the manufacturers of the medications mentioned.

Printed in the United States of America

First Edition 1984

Library of Congress Cataloging in Publication Data

Rayburn, William F.
   Obstetrics for the house officer.

   (The House officer series)
   Includes bibliographies and index.
   1. Obstetrics—Handbooks, manuals, etc.   I. Lavin, Justin P.   II. Title.   III. Series.
[DNLM: 1. Obstetrics—handbooks.   2. Pregnancy Complications—handbooks.
WQ 39 R265o]
RG531.R38   1988   618.2   87-34609
ISBN 0-683-07159-9

88 89 90 91
1 2 3 4 5 6 7 8 9 10

Preface

Every pregnant woman and her unborn infant deserve optimal care before, during, and after delivery. Because of improved fetal surveillance techniques and more successful management of certain obstetric and medical complications, many options are now available in providing appropriate care. Good clinical judgment is essential in individualizing patient care, and current advances in perinatal medicine must be kept in proper perspective.

This manual is intended to provide guidelines to the house officer on how, when, and where to appropriately handle routine and uncommon clinical conditions. Protocols used at the University of Nebraska Medical Center and Akron City Hospital are presented in dealing with such problems encountered during pregnancy. Statements in this book are meant to be guidelines, since each hospital should develop its own protocol for managing complicated pregnancies.

Information was gathered from a review of the current literature, discussions with respected colleagues, and our own clinical impressions. The number of references has been restricted to limit the size of the book. The peer review journal articles listed in the "suggested reading" section at the end of each chapter are among the best by well regarded researchers and have been discussed at our frequent journal club meetings.

We wish to thank the faculty members within our departments of obstetrics and gynecology for their critical review of these guidelines. Rebecca Christensen and Michael Schneider were especially helpful in their review from a house officer's perspective. Special thanks is also expressed to Gretta Friedrich and Valerie Owens who worked closely with us in preparing this second edition.

William F. Rayburn, M.D.
Omaha

Justin P. Lavin, M.D.
Akron

Contents

Chapter 1

Prenatal Care

Gestational Age Determination

Along with counseling the patient in preparing for childbirth, accurate dating of the pregnancy is essential for timing of a repeat cesarean section, assessment of fetal growth (large or small for gestational age), decision making if pregnancy intervention is planned, timing of an amniocentesis (genetic, fetal lung maturity testing), intrauterine transfusion, assessment of multifetal gestation, avoiding iatrogenic premature delivery, and predicting neonatal survival if preterm delivery is anticipated. Accuracy in predicting the delivery date is improved by combining the methods described below and documenting these landmarks on the prenatal record.

Methods

Last Menstrual Period
If known with certainty, it is the most reliable clinical estimator of gestational age. However, dating is uncertain in 14-58% (average 40%) of all pregnancies. Reasons include patient recall inability, inaccurate reporting, first trimester bleeding, oligomenorrhea, recent pregnancy, and breast feeding. Menstrual dating requires a history of any contraceptive method (particularly oral contraceptives) and any menstrual irregularities.

Initial Positive Pregnancy Test
Present methods for measuring human chorionic gonadotropin (hCG) and the earliest time for accurate measurements are listed in Table 1.1.

Initial Uterine Examination
Uterine size may be larger than dates in the presence of a full bladder, trophoblastic disease, uterine fibroids, and twins.

Initial Fetal Heart Auscultation
With amplified (Doppler) auscultation, the fetal heart sounds should be heard by 12 weeks or sooner, depending on whether the uterus is pushed up out of the pelvis by a full bladder. Unamplified heart sounds are usually heard by 20 weeks.

Table 1.1
Pregnancy Tests

Method	Detectable (+) result (postconception)	Test sensitivity mIU/ml
Immunoassay		
Hemagglutination inhibition*	3-4 weeks	750-3500
Enzyme immunoassay	2 weeks	25(serum)-50(urine)
Radioreceptor assay (RRA)	2-3 weeks	100-200
Radioimmunoassay (RIA)		
Rapid, qualitative	2 weeks	20-40
24-48 hr, quantitative	1 week	2-4

*Examples include Pregnosticon, UCG, DAP, Pregnosis, Gravindex.

Initial Perception of Fetal Movement
        A primigravid patient usually perceives light fetal movements by 19-20 weeks, whereas a multigravid patient often feels motion by 17-18 weeks. This parameter is often inexact.

Serial Uterine Fundal Height Examinations
        An excellent correlation exists between fundal height measurement (in centimeters) from the upper symphysis to fundus and gestational age (in weeks) between 18-30 weeks. This measurement is influenced by the patient's obesity, fetal position, differences between examiners, and an empty or full bladder.

Estimated Fetal Weight
        Although often inexact ($\pm$ 500 gm), the recording of an estimation of fetal weight is recommended during each clinic visit in the third trimester of pregnancy. Suspecting a large fetus at term is especially important.

Ultrasonography
        A recent National Institutes of Health (NIH) consensus committee concluded that at the present time, there are insufficient data available to establish the cost effectiveness of routine ultrasound examination in pregnancy. On the other hand, that group suggested that ultrasound should be performed to confirm pregnancy dating if the historical dates are in question, if obstetrical intervention or elective delivery is likely to be required, or if a size-date discrepancy exists.
        Early anatomic landmarks include measurements of the gestational sac between 6-10 weeks and crown-rump between 7-13 weeks. The diameter of the gestational sac is 2 cm at 6 weeks and 5 cm at 10 weeks. The crown-rump length (CRL) in centimeters plus 6.5 approximates the

estimated gestational age. For example, a CRL of 5.5 cm should correspond to a gestational age of 12 weeks.
Beyond the 13th week, the most accurate assessment is obtained by averaging biparietal diameter (BPD), cerebellum diameter, head circumference, abdominal circumference and femur length measurements. Table 1.2 lists these sonographic measurements for the corresponding gestational age. This correlation is less accurate with advancing gestation.

Table 1.2
Sonographic Measurements and Gestational Age Determinations

Weeks Gestation	BPD (cm)	Cerebellum Diameters (cm)	Head Circumf. (cm)	Abdominal Circumf. (cm)	Femur Length (cm)
12			6.7	5.7	1.0
13			8.2	6.7	1.3
14	2.8		9.6	8.1	1.6
15	3.2	1.4	11.0	9.3	1.9
16	3.6	1.6	12.4	10.5	2.2
17	3.9	1.7	13.7	11.6	2.5
18	4.2	1.8	15.0	12.8	2.8
19	4.5	1.9	16.2	14.0	3.2
20	4.8	2.0	17.4	15.1	3.5
21	5.1	2.2	18.6	16.2	3.8
22	5.4	2.3	19.8	17.3	4.0
23	5.8	2.4	20.9	18.4	5.8
24	6.1	2.5	22.0	19.5	4.4
25	6.4	2.8	23.0	20.6	4.6
26	6.7	2.9	24.0	21.6	4.8
27	7.0	3.0	25.0	22.7	5.0
28	7.2	3.1	25.9	23.9	5.3
29	7.5	3.4	26.8	24.8	5.5
30	7.8	3.5	27.7	25.8	5.7
31	8.0	3.8	28.6	26.8	6.0
32	8.2	3.9	29.4	27.8	6.2
33	8.5	4.0	30.1	28.7	6.4
34	8.7	4.0	30.0	29.7	6.6
35	8.8	4.1	31.5	30.7	6.8
36	9.0	4.3	32.2	31.6	7.1
37	9.2	4.5	32.8	32.5	7.3
38	9.3	4.9	33.4	33.4	7.5
39	9.4	5.2	34.0	34.4	7.7
40	9.5		34.5	35.2	8.0
41			35.0	36.1	
42			35.4	37.0	

*All fetal growth measurements correspond to the 50th percentile for that gestational age.

Other
    Biochemical tests such as hCG, human placental lactogen, and
alpha-fetoprotein determinations are not considered accurate predictors
of gestational age.   X-rays of the fetal skeleton may be seen in 1/3
cases by 20 weeks, 1/2 cases by 24 weeks, and all by 28 weeks.   A
distal femoral epiphysis is usually observed by 36 weeks. However, x-
rays are much less accurate than ultrasound and carry the risk of
exposure to ionizing radiation.   Therefore, they should rarely if ever
be utilized for pregnancy dating.

Recommendations to Patients

    The following are general recommendations for patients as they
seek prenatal care.   These patient instructions are divided into three
major categories: symptoms experienced during pregnancy, precautions to
take during pregnancy, and preparing to care for the infant after
delivery.

Symptoms during Pregnancy

    Nausea is an expected and common symptom, especially during early
pregnancy.   Although often distressing, it is a normal and favorable
sign of a healthy pregnancy.   Nausea results from the altered
circulating blood hormone levels.   A handout should be available to
provide appropriate recommendations for diet that should help relieve
symptoms.   However, knowing that nausea and even vomiting are favorable
signs, the patient may be able to handle these symptoms without medical
intervention.   Simple nausea is often treated expectantly with
reassurance and diet manipulation.   Prenatal vitamins, antihistamines,
or both may be helpful.
    Persistent **vomiting** requires stronger antiemetic therapy to avoid
maternal dehydration, weight loss, and electrolyte imbalance.
Phenothiazines, notably promethazine (Phenergan), are used commonly and
with safety.   Less is known about the use of metoclopramide or
transdermal scopolamine.   If conservative therapy and antiemetic drugs
are inadequate, hospitalization may be necessary.   Enteral fluid and
nutrient therapy (especially parenteral nutrient therapy) are being
considered as more becomes known about effectiveness and safety.
    Breast tenderness is another frequent symptom that occurs early in
pregnancy, often before the first missed period.   This also is related
to the increased circulating hormone levels.   All throughout the
pregnancy the breasts are preparing themselves for lactation and milk
production.   The degree of tenderness is variable but may be influenced
by temperature changes, being worse during cold weather.   Lactation is
common later in gestation and should not be alarming.   In addition,
sexual stimulation may increase the tenderness of the breasts; however,
this is not harmful and sexual activity should not be curtailed because
of the changes in the breasts.   We do recommend that the patient wear a
well-supporting, well-fitting bra, especially if she is physically
active. The cup size of the bra is expected to increase as much as two

sizes during pregnancy. Nursing bras are available and may be worn later in pregnancy.

Profound **fatigue** can be expected, particularly during the first and last trimesters. The body is expending a tremendous amount of energy in the establishment of a normal pregnancy, and fatigue should cause no great concern. Daily rest with frequent naps and proper nutrition are necessary during this period. In addition, a daily routine of exercise, such as walking, swimming, or bicycling, is recommended.

Weight gain is a concern of all patients and is an indirect guide for nutrition and pregnancy well-being. It is recommended that weight gain be no less than 20 pounds. Some may gain as much as 40 pounds, and this will occur without any apparent complications. Weight loss or dietary restrictions during pregnancy must be avoided. A gain of more than 2 pounds per week suggests the possibility of fluid retention. Good **nutrition** does not necessarily mean eating excessively. Several small snacks or three well-balanced meals per day and a late night snack are recommended. Since the fetus can gain up to 1/2 pound per week in the last few months of pregnancy, the appetite and dietary habits may change.

Back **pain,** pelvic pain, and even leg pain are common, especially in late pregnancy. As additional weight is carried, the ligaments holding the pelvis together are softening in anticipation of childbirth. For the most part, these discomforts are normal, and lying on the side or a change in posture will usually give relief. Persistent back pain should be sought, since this may suggest an infection in the kidneys or bladder or even premature labor.

A collection of extra water or **edema** may occur in the feet and the legs. This is common during pregnancy, especially after standing or sitting for long periods. This normally occurs from increased blood pooling in the leg veins, because the pregnancy hormones soften and dilate the blood vessel walls. Support pantyhose may be worn while working and standing erect. Knee-hose and garters should be avoided, because they further constrict the blood supply returning from the feet and lower legs. It is important to note whether any rings become tight and difficult to remove or if there is any swelling of your face, particularly in the morning. "Fluid pills," water pills, or diuretics should rarely be given during pregnancy, because they can decrease the blood volume and blood flow to the uterus and fetus.

Urinary frequency is one of the earliest signs of pregnancy. Going to the bathroom nearly twice as frequently is common, and is most noticeable during the first and last trimesters from increased pressure on the bladder. Since the kidneys function best at night while the patient is lying on her side, she should expect to awaken several times to empty her bladder. Should she experience any burning or pain in the bladder area or the back, a urinary tract infection may be present. This should be reported immediately, since if not adequately treated, a serious infection of the kidneys may develop.

During pregnancy the amount of blood increases dramatically. A symptom of this may be **nasal congestion** that can cause difficulty in breathing and even nausea. Decongestants and antihistamines are used frequently. Bleeding of the nose may occasionally accompany nasal congestion. This may be worse during winter because of dry air in heated buildings. Placing Vaseline on the inner aspect of each nostril before going to bed will help.

Changes during pregnancy occur in the stomach and intestines that will result in more efficient absorption of food. One of these changes is increased acid secretion by the stomach, and this can result in **heartburn.** If prone to heartburn, the patient should avoid smoking, drinking caffeinated beverages, and lying down after a meal. At night the entire head of the bed (not just her head) should be elevated at least 3 inches. This can be done by placing a brick or other suitable object under the frame of the bed. Antacids, such as Tums, Maalox, Mylanta, and Amphojel, may be taken up to every 2 hours if the above measures are unsuccessful.

Constipation is experienced by many patients during all stages of pregnancy. This is due in part to the iron content of vitamin pills, absorption of more fluids into the bloodstream, and compression of the bowel by the enlargening uterus. Constipation will be helped by increasing fluid intake to three or more glasses of water or milk each day. We also recommend eating high-fiber foods, such as bran cereal and fresh fruit. Stool softeners are not recommended routinely, but cellulose powders (Metamucil) may be taken without harm.

Hemorrhoids may occur during pregnancy (particularly after delivery) due to the softening of tissues including the blood vessels and the increase in the circulating blood volume. These rarely require surgery and will usually subside after delivery. Preparation H, Anusol, or Tucks may be used without concern to decrease the swelling and relieve the pain. In addition, a cold compress will often help.

Although the choice of **clothes** is a personal matter, those worn before pregnancy will become very tight and uncomfortable. It is important that garments be loose fitting and comfortable. In addition, shoes should be comfortable, allowing for the modest swelling that is a normal symptom of pregnancy, and be of a style that provides stability and prevents trips or falls.

An increase in the amount of **vaginal discharge** is a normal expected symptom of early and late pregnancy and does not require any therapy. The increased circulating blood hormones result in a thickening of the vaginal tissues and an increase in the discharge from the cervix. Pregnancy can also predispose to yeast infections (Monilia or Candida). This may result in a further increase in the vaginal discharge, a change in its color or odor, and a staining or crusting on undergarments or itching on the lips of the vagina. Should these symptoms occur, the physician should prescribe the appropriate therapy. We discourage douching during pregnancy.

Precautions to Take during Pregnancy

A proper **diet** is essential to good health during pregnancy. We recommend fresh fruit, fresh vegetables, lean meats (chicken, fish), and low-fat dairy products. Intolerance to milk is common during pregnancy and may cause heartburn and induce cramping, diarrhea, and even excessive gas formation. It is acceptable to substitute cheese or yogurt or add chocolate to the milk. Most doctors prescribe prenatal **vitamin** supplements, but they are not essential during pregnancy as long as nutrition is adequate. The value of fluoride tablets during pregnancy remains to be seen but may be associated with a lower risk of dental caries in the child's primary teeth. The fluoride content in most water supplies is usually sufficient. Iron supplementation is necessary, in that the developing blood cells of the infant will take away more iron than the mother's body can absorb from diet during the nine-month period. Therefore, a prenatal vitamin containing iron or an iron tablet alone needs to be taken daily during pregnancy and lactation. Fast foods, though economical and easily available, should be discouraged as a staple part of the diet because they contain excess fat, salt, sugar, etc. For the same reason, "junk foods" should be avoided in general. Caffeinated beverages, such as colas, tea, and coffee, should be ingested in moderation during pregnancy (two or less servings per day). A list of foods in any special diet (example, vegetarian diet) should be sought.

In our experience many patients have taken **drugs** before or during the early stages of pregnancy. Any drugs taken before pregnancy, during early pregnancy, or throughout pregnancy should be sought. Those prescribed for a medical illness (hypertension, diabetes, epilepsy, heart disease, asthma) may still be necessary and should be taken.

Smoking during pregnancy is discouraged, as is being in a smoke-filled room for any prolonged period. There are many studies indicating that infants born of mothers who smoke have gained an average of 200 gm (5 oz) less than babies born of nonsmoking mothers. In addition, nicotine from cigarettes is concentrated in the breast tissue and will be stored there to be delivered in the milk. Nicotine absorbed from the milk by the breastfeeding baby can cause symptoms that are undesirable. If the patient is unable to quit, we strongly recommend that she smoke less than 1/2 pack per day and that the cigarettes contain the lowest tar and nicotine content. Adverse effects of marijuana on the fetus are being studied at this time and are not as well understood as those caused by some other drugs. Any street drugs (LSD, "uppers," "downers," cocaine, "angel dust") are strongly discouraged during pregnancy, since all have been shown to have adverse effects on the developing infant.

Many patients will be concerned about an alcoholic drink taken during the early stages of your pregnancy. There is no absolute safe level of ingestion of **alcohol** during pregnancy. However, signs of the fetal alcohol syndrome require excessive consumption (five or more hard drinks per day) for prolonged periods of time. An occasional alcoholic beverage, such as a glass of wine, beer, or a mixed drink, may be ingested without probable concern.

Sex should not be discontinued during pregnancy. The anticipation of a new family member may result in an increase in normal sexual desires. As pregnancy progresses, sexual activity becomes more difficult, more tiring, and sometimes uncomfortable. However, there is no reason to discontinue sexual activity because it is generally believed not to pose any risk to the fetus or to result in an increased risk of premature labor or delivery. Orgasm will frequently cause a uterine contraction, which may be painful but does no apparent harm. On the other hand, if she experiences any signs of an abnormal discharge, any recent vaginal bleeding, or any leakage of fluid from the vagina, abstaining from sexual activity would seem appropriate. In addition, a history of a "weak" or incompetent cervix, premature labor, or an untreated infection should be sought. The mucus in the cervix during a normal pregnancy forms an effective plug such that the ejaculate remains in the vagina and does not gain access to the uterus.

The patient should refrain from using very hot water while **bathing**. The water is too hot if it reddens the skin. In addition, precautions should be taken in getting in and out of the tub. As pregnancy progresses, it may be important to have an attendant available. It is common to become very lightheaded, particulary late in pregnancy, particularly when changing positions from lying down to standing, sitting to standing, and getting out of the bath tub. Sitting in a sauna bath or hot tub with water temperature higher than 110o should be avoided or at least not continued for more than 10 minutes. The heat can result in an increase in the core body temperature that may be damaging to your developing fetus.

Pregnancy induces changes in the gums and teeth, and **dental care** is encouraged during pregnancy. Major procedures that require much manipulation or surgery should be discussed beforehand. Most dentists are very cautious about performing any dental procedure during the first and last few months of pregnancy. If dental x-rays are necessary, the dentist should provide a protective apron that shields the fetus from any x-ray exposure.

Exercise should be encouraged during pregnancy. Specific exercises in preparation for childbirth will be taught during childbirth classes. However, until these classes begin, daily walks are to be encouraged. If facilities are available, swimming and bicycling are also excellent during pregnancy. More programmed exercising to be sought include aerobics dancing, jogging, skating, weight lifting, etc. Jogging may be continued during pregnancy for those persons already in good shape. Uterine contractility is not thought to increase with moderate exercise, and any fetal heart rate changes are uncommon and thought to be transient in an otherwise uncomplicated pregnancy. Exercising may be continued throughout pregnancy; however, strenuous exercise should be decreased during the latter half of the pregnancy. Should there be a medical complication (high blood pressure, diabetes), the patient should abstain from vigorous exercise. Following an exercise period, the patient should program a time in which she lies on her side (preferably left side) for a minimum of 1 hour each day. This has been shown to improve the circulation to the uterus and fetus and it also assists the uterus to relax.

During the initial prenatal visit time is allowed to discuss the **recurrence of any prior pregnancy complications**. General risk figures are relatively encouraging and often helpful for patient education. The data are usually derived from large groups of heterogeneous pregnancies and may have been gathered in a biased way. The etiology is also often obscure and likely to remain so. An honest appraisal of the chances of success in any future pregnancy is necessary for patient support. Table 1.3 indicates recurrence risk figures for the most severe complications of prior pregnancies.

Table 1.3
Recurrence Risks for Common Pregnancy Complications

Previous Complication	Recurrence Risk	
Hydatidiform mole	1.3-2.9%	
Recurrent miscarriage	20-30%	
Ectopic pregnancy	50%	involuntary infertility
	35-40%	successful pregnancy
	10-15%	recurrent ectopic
Mild preeclampsia	2.0%	for severe preeclampsia
	29.0%	for mild preeclampsia
Severe preeclampsia	7.5%	for severe preeclampsia
	30.0%	for mild preeclampsia
Placental abruption	15%	
Preterm labor x 1	15%	
x 2	30%	
Gestational diabetes	25-75%	

Only 6% of births in the United States are among women **age 35** or older. These women often postpone beginning a family until their education has been completed and a career has been started. There appears to be a greater risk of spontaneous abortion, and the stillbirth rate seems to double by the late 30's and increases to three- to four-fold by the mid 40's. Chromosomal abnormalities, especially trisomies 13, 18, and 21, and sex chromosome aneuploidies increase logarithmically with maternal age starting in the 30's. Genetic counseling should therefore be offered to any expectant mothers who are 35 or older. Bleeding from a placenta previa or abruptio placenta is also thought to be more common in late gestation in older patients. Hypertension, preeclampsia, and diabetes are not only more common but seem to carry an even greater risk for older women, resulting more frequently in fetal demise. There also appear to be more problems with abnormal labor patterns and a higher incidence of cesarean section.

An **amniocentesis** (sampling of the fluid around the baby) may be done early in pregnancy for genetic reasons or before delivery to determine that the baby's lungs are mature. A sonogram is usually performed beforehand to localize the placenta and vital fetal parts. Every attempt will be made to avoid these vital structures, and the risk to the fetus is very low (only one in 250-500 cases shows signs of infection, bleeding, or fetal death).

Ultrasonography to look at the fetus is performed often but is not a routine procedure. There must be an adequate indication; to perform the test merely because of the patient's curiosity is unjustified. We avoid ultrasound exposure during the first few months of pregnancy until the baby's organs are better formed. However, a scan is performed if a complication (example, vaginal bleeding) occurs during the first few months of pregnancy. The energy of sound waves transmitted from the machine is very low, and no human study has indicated that this procedure is unsafe.

Travel late in pregnancy should be discussed. As a general rule, we discourage long trips within the last month, particularly within the last two weeks of pregnancy or when a complication has occurred. If there are situations that will require travel late in pregnancy, the following are necessary: a vaginal examination before leaving to determine the dilation of the cervix and the name of a competent obstetrician in the community to be visited. If travel is by automobile, one stop is recommended at least every 2 hours. During this travel break, which should be from 10-15 minutes, it is necessary to walk and empty the bladder. It is safe to fly during pregnancy, and there is no increased risk of miscarriage or anomalies to the fetus.

Vaginal bleeding at any time during pregnancy should be reported. It is not uncommon for slight spotting to occur after sex or a pelvic examination. However, this should be reported if it persists.

Uterine contractions within 2 months before the "due date" are common but should be reported. Irregular contractions occurring less frequently than every 8 min are particularly common and are probably Braxton-Hicks contractions. The physician should be notified if these persist and are as frequent as every 5 minutes.

Approximately 1% of all pregnant women are exposed to abdominal **x-rays** during the first trimester. Radiation exposures usually result in doses much less than 5 rads, and the resulting risks are usually small compared with other risks of pregnancy. A dose of about 10 rads is the lowest amount associated with structural embryonic or fetal defects. After fertilization, radiation effects are likely to be "all or none" during tubal transport, and the embryo after implantation may be more resistant to the lethal effects of radiation. X-rays should generally be avoided during pregnancy. Should these be necessary (such as a chest x-ray or abdominal film), we encourage shielding the uterus. In doing so, we feel that these necessary x-rays are quite safe. On occasion, a patient will report that an x-ray was performed very early in pregnancy when pregnancy was unsuspected. Any risk to the fetus is highly unlikely, and there is no indication for a therapeutic abortion. We have not yet seen an unfavorable pregnancy outcome because of a diagnostic x-ray alone.

Fevers of 100° F or greater should also be reported. This may be due to a flu-like illness but may also represent a more serious infection such as a kidney infection or pneumonia. The actual harm to the fetus from high fevers cannot be clearly determined.

Prior **venereal infections** (especially gonorrhea, syphilis, herpes, and Chlamydia) should be reported. Further tests may be necessary to determine whether an infection is still present and active.

Severe, continuous **headaches** are uncommon during pregnancy and should be reported. Persistent headaches associated with high blood pressure are often accompanied with dimming and blurring of vision and spots seen before the eyes.

Severe or persistent **abdominal pain** or cramping may be associated with a placental separation from the uterine wall (abruptio placenta) or premature labor. These pains, are often sharp and well localized. On the other hand, it is not uncommon to have occasional abdominal cramps that are related to Braxton-Hicks uterine contractions. The patient should remain at rest and notify her physician if the cramping persists.

A sudden escape of clear **fluid from the vagina** indicates either a loss of urine or a rupture of the bag of water. It is often difficult to distinguish between the two, and the physician should be notified to arrange an examination. This problem usually occurs within the last 2 months of pregnancy.

A decrease in fetal movement is a common patient concern. We have fetal activity charts available for patients who have a pregnancy complication or notice a decrease in fetal movement. A patient is asked to keep a daily record of the baby's activity during at least one convenient hour of monitoring while lying on her side. Documented **fetal inactivity** suggests distress and requires further evaluation.

Blood pressure changes can be monitored both in the clinic and at home. For patients with a prior history of **high blood pressure** or kidney disease, we frequently ask that they purchase a blood pressure cuff and stethoscope at their local drug store or medical supply house. By monitoring the blood pressure at home as well as in the clinic, we have a better idea of the degree of the problem and can better counsel the patient.

We see many patients who have **diabetes** complicating the pregnancy. Along with checking blood sugars in the clinic, we usually have our patients check them at home. Machines to monitor blood sugar levels are available at many pharmacies for use at home, and charts are provided to record the results.

Preparing for Childbirth and Infant Care

Specific information about **childbirth classes** is available in the clinic. We strongly encourage our patients to prepare for labor by attending these classes even if a repeat cesarean section will be undertaken. If there are any concerns about **delivery,** discuss these with the patient and any other doctor who is likely to perform the delivery. Also discuss what to expect during labor and delivery, and what may be used for **pain relief.** If necessary, discuss with her the possibility or probability of needing a cesarean delivery.

Cesarean section classes are available if the patient has an interest in learning more about the surgery. A **prior cesarean section** does not necessarily require a repeat cesarean section. Every effort can be made to allow a vaginal birth experience if the patient and her spouse desire.

Information should be provided about various **options available** during the course of labor and delivery. These options include an intravenous line to be maintained throughout labor, electronic fetal heart monitoring, vaginal prep, sibling visitation, 24-hour rooming-in, early hospital discharge, and visiting nurse home visits. Most hospitals are now providing rooms in which the mother can both labor and deliver. Such a "birthing room" may decrease the admission-to-delivery interval, decrease the analgesia requirement, allow more freedom of movement, require less suturing, increase rooming-in time, and decrease hospital costs. State law requires that each infant receive silver nitrate, erythromycin, or tetracycline in its eyes to guard against gonorrhea. This will be performed routinely unless the parents voice strong reservations.

If desired, a **circumcision** is performed within the first few days after the baby boy is delivered. We strongly encourage that you seek her thoughts on circumcision before labor. Information about pros and cons of circumcision should be available from the clinic. This is a surgical procedure, and although the complication rate is very low, a circumcision is cosmetic and not medically necessary.

Although it is not necessary to visit the **baby's doctor** before delivery, we do encourage a pediatrician or family physician to be chosen beforehand. It is not necessary for that doctor to attend the delivery or see the baby shortly after delivery. If the baby's doctor has practice privileges at the hospital, the nurses in the nursery will call his (her) office. The baby's first visit should be scheduled usually within the first month after delivery.

Baby furniture such as a crib and dresser should be purchased before delivery. There are many products available and the parents may wish to discuss these items with a physician or nurse during the antepartum visits. It is a law in many states that the baby leave the hospital in a safety-approved car seat.

We are often surprised that many patients have not chosen a **baby's name** before birth. This can be an anxiety-provoking situation, and we encourage selection before birth.

Several methods are available to determine the **baby's sex** before delivery, but these require an expensive and potentially hazardous procedure (amniocentesis) to measure hormone levels or look at genetic chromosomes. During the ultrasound examination, we can often determine the fetal sex by looking for a penis. This is not altogether accurate, and an ultrasound performed only for determining the baby's sex is unjustified.

It may be possible after delivery for the new mother to have a private room with her baby. Although this cannot be guaranteed, it is possible to have **rooming-in** privileges. We strongly encourage that friends and family members abide by **visiting hours** in the postpartum area. The husband or identified primary visitor may visit at any time after the delivery. More specific information about sibling visits in the mother's room will be provided on request.

Proper nutrition and continuing the iron or vitamins are necessary for the first 2 months after delivery. **Exercises** to promote support of the abdmonial muscles may begin immediately after a vaginal delivery. Overstrenuous exercise is to be discouraged, however, during the initial 2 weeks. After a cesarean section, exercises are to be avoided until she sees her doctor 2 weeks after delivery.

Family visits at home should be well planned, especially with the intent of allowing the patient to relax. Even though this is an exciting time, be aware that the new parents may have an emotional letdown because of a disruption of the normal routine, a lack of sleep, or reduced attention from the spouse.

Sexual intercourse may be resumed at any time after delivery. Vaginal pain may be present in breastfeeding mothers or from episiotomy discomfort. **Birth control** should be discussed again before discharge. A diaphragm cannot be fitted until the uterus is normal size (usually 6 or more weeks after delivery). Although ovulation does not occur in the first month, it is possible to become pregnant before the next clinic visit, so foam and condoms should be used. Women who are breastfeeding require contraception also.

Outpatient Laboratory Tests

The first prenatal visit should include the following tests: blood type, blood Rh, antibody screen, complete blood count, rubella titer, urinalysis, Testuria, serologic test for syphilis (VDRL or rapid plasma reagin (RPR)), Pap smear, and tuberculin skin test. Maternal serum alpha-fetoprotein screening should be discussed and, if the patient desires, should be undertaken between the 14th-18th weeks. At the beginning of the third trimester (24-28 weeks), the following tests should be performed routinely: complete blood count, 1-hr post 50 gm glucola glucose determination, and antibody screen (if Rh negative and unsensitized). Other tests to be ordered under special conditions are shown in Table 1.4.

Table 1.4
Indications for Special Tests during Pregnancy

Special Test	Indications
Gonorrhea culture	Prior venereal infection, vaginitis, drug abuser, adolescent; may be required routinely in certain states
Clean-catch urine for culture	Patients with consecutive positive Testurias, symptoms strongly suggestive of urinary tract infection, or prior history of renal disease

Table 1.4 (Continued)

Special Test	Indications
Herpes culture	Vulvar lesion, prior infection, recent exposure
HIV antibody for AIDS	Patients at increased risk to be exposed to the AIDS virus, i.e., intravenous drug abusers, prostitutes, hemophiliacs, and gravidas whose sexual partners may be at increased risk because of the above factors or homosexual activity. Informed consent should be obtained prior to testing because of the potential adverse psychosocial implications of a positive result.
Shielded chest x-ray	Positive tuberculin skin test, significant past or present respiratory or cardiac illness
Ultrasound	Uncertain menstrual dates, uterine size disparity, prior cesarean section, medical or obstetric complications, poor obstetric history
1-hour post 50 gm glucola glucose determinations (before 28th week)	Family history of diabetes, prior macrosomic fetus, prior poor obstetric history, persistent glycosuria, suspected polyhydramnios, maternal age 35 or older, obesity, recurrent moniliasis, or prior anomalous infant.
Hemoglobin A_{1C}	Maternal diabetes or prior macrosomic infant
Rubella titer (later in pregnancy)	If prior titer was 1:8-1:16 or suspected exposure to rubella if titer less than 1:16
Paternal blood typing	Rh negative mother-to-be Uncertainty of father-to-be

Drug Effects on the Fetus

With the increased awareness of drug effects on the unborn infant, there is a general reluctance by patients to take drugs during pregnancy. Despite this trend, the average pregnant patient takes two drugs, besides iron or vitamin supplements, before labor. This number of drugs actually increases rather than decreases as gestation progresses, and approximately one-half of these drugs are over-the-counter preparations (aspirin, acetaminophen, decongestants).

The initial prenatal examination should include a history of any prescribed or nonprescription drugs taken at conception, during the first trimester, or presently. The most common drugs taken at conception and during early pregnancy include oral contraceptives and diet pills (many of which are amphetamines or amphetamine-like compounds).

Most drugs have no apparent adverse effect on the fetus. Drugs or chemicals account for no more than 1% of all major malformations, while multifactorial or unknown causes are implicated in two-thirds of all human malformations. Teratogenic effects include not only obvious malformations or abortions but also involve altered fetal growth, carcinogenesis, functional deficits, or mutagenesis. Therefore, no drug can be considered absolutely safe to use during pregnacy.

Our limited knowledge about specific drugs is gathered from case reports, epidemiologic studies, or animal studies. Differing experimental animal species are usually exposed to high drug doses during early fetal development. The few drugs with known teratogenic effects include anticonvulsants, coumadin, alcohol, folic acid antagonists (methotrexate, aminopterin), diethylstilbestrol, androgens, and thalidomide (Table 1.5). Fortunately, those drugs with known or suspected teratogenic effects, except phenytoin, are unnecessary during pregnancy. Suspected teratogenic drugs include alkylating agents, nicotine, sulfonylureas, cis-retinoic acid, valproic acid, and benzodiazepines. Their effects are also listed in Table 1.5. These drugs are also not needed during pregnancy.

General Recommendations

The overall incidence of birth defects in the general population is 2-4%. Most drugs pose no obvious threat to the fetus, but added risks relate to the dose, duration, any drug metabolites, and gestational age at the time of exposure. The genotype of the mother and fetus and the effect from any other drugs must also be considered.

Accurate dating of gestational age is necessary when a patient expresses concern about drug exposure during early pregnancy. The drug or chemical may have been taken before implantation or after organogenesis. Unless absolutely necessary, all drugs should be avoided during the first trimester.

An amniocentesis to screen for drug or metabolite levels is not recommended. A maternal serum alpha-fetoprotein level between 14-20 weeks may be helpful, especially when a drug such as valproic acid, which is thought to be associated with an increased risk of open neural tube defects, has been taken. Ultrasonography is useful for dating a gestation, searching for major malformations, and assessing fetal growth. Reassuring findings do not guarantee a "normal" fetus, however.

Table 1.5
Drugs with Known or Suspected Teratogenic Effects

Drug	Teratogenic Effect
Known teratogens	
Anticonvulsants Trimethadione, phenytoin	Facial dysmorphogenesis, mild mental retardation, growth retardation
Anticoagulants Coumadin and congeners	Nasal hypoplasia, epiphyseal stippling, optic atrophy, mental retardation
Alcohol	Fetal alcohol syndrome - growth retardation, mild mental retardation, increase in anomalies
Folic acid antagonists Methotrexate, aminopterin	Abortion, multiple malformations
Hormones Diethylstilbestrol and congeners	Vaginal adenosis, carcinogenesis, cervical and uterine anomalies, epididymal abnormalities
Androgens	Masculinization of female fetus
Methyl mercury	CNS damage, growth retardation
Thalidomide	Phocomelia
Valproic acid	Open neural tube defects
Cis-retinoic acid	Hydrocephalus, cardiac defects, ear and hearing defects
Suspected teratogens	
Alkylating agents	Abortion, anomalies
Hormones Oral contraceptives	Limb reduction and cardiac defects (?)
Progestins	Limb reduction and cardiac defects (?)
Lithium carbonate	Ebstein's anomaly
Nicotine	Growth delay
Sulfonylureas	Anomalies (?)
Benzodiazepines	Facial clefts (?)

The risks and benefits must be considered when prescribed medication is necessary to treat any underlying medical or obstetric complication. As a general rule, perinatal outcomes are more favorable with the appropriate selection of a drug(s) to treat any underlying medical disorder. Even though the lowest effective doses are desired, serum concentrations of such prescription drugs as phenobarbital, phenytoin, aminophylline, or digoxin decrease during pregnancy. Therefore, increased doses of these medications are required to maintain adequate therapeutic levels.

Specific Drugs

Mild Analgesics

No conclusive evidence exists in humans that aspirin causes fetal malformations. Salicylates may inhibit prostaglandin synthesis and reduce platelet aggregation properties. Gestation and labor may be prolonged if large doses have been taken. Prolonged bleeding time even with small doses may last for 5-7 days and may increase blood loss at delivery.

Salicylates cross the placenta freely, and premature closure of the ductus arteriosus is theoretically possible. This event may cause pulmonary arterial hypertension and cardiopulmonary complications in the newborn. Other potential fetal or neonatal problems include an increased bleeding time and jaundice from competition with bilirubin for albumin binding.

Because of these potentially harmful effects in the third trimester, it is preferable to avoid aspirin use and to substitute acetaminophen if necessary. Acetaminophen has similar analgesic and antipyretic properties, which may result from prostaglandin synthetase inhibition or direct hypothalamic stimulation. To the best of our knowledge, no consistent information has revealed any detrimental effects of acetaminophen on the fetus when used in the usual therapeutic doses. However, further clinical or epidemiologic studies are necessary.

Decongestants and Antihistamines

Physiologic nasal congestion, upper respiratory viral infections, and allergic symptoms are common during pregnancy and frequently require decongestant or antihistamine therapy. The pseudoephedrine-containing decongestants have not been shown to be teratogenic in human fetuses. Animal studies suggest a greater likelihood of diminished uteroplacental perfusion, which may affect fetal acid-base balance. Persons with hypertension may wish to avoid the use of the medicines during pregnancy.

Compared with a group of pregnant patients who took no drugs, no increased incidence of congenital anomalies has been reported in patients using such antihistamines as brompheniramine, chlorpheniramine, and meclizine. Antihistamines and decongestants are excreted in breast milk, but neonatal effects are not considered significant in the usual dosages.

Antacids

Over-the-counter antacid preparations contain either aluminum hydroxide, calcium carbonate, sodium bicarbonate, or magnesium hydroxide. Antacid use is most common in late pregnancy for relief of heartburn from gastric hyperacidity. It is considered safe, unless high doses are ingested chronically. Sodium within certain antacids

(Alka-Seltzer, Rolaids, Bromo-Seltzer) should be avoided when excess fluid retention or toxemia is present. Adverse effects from antacid use include constipation and impaired absorption of such drugs as tetracyclines, cephalosporins, and chlorpromazine. Although absorbed calcium or magnesium from within these preparations may cross the placenta or be excreted in breast milk, effects on the fetus or neonate are not considered to be significant.

Penicillins

Penicillins are commonly prescribed during pregnancy for treatment of urinary tract or upper respiratory infections. To achieve serum drug concentrations similar to those in the nonpregnant state, large or more frequent dosages may be necessary. Most studies have failed to show adverse effects of penicillins on the developing fetus. They may therefore be considered safe to use in nonallergic patients. Penicillins will appear in breast milk and may cause diarrhea and candidiasis in the nursing infant with prolonged exposure.

Marijuana

Marijuana smoking during pregnancy is to be discouraged. The active ingredient, tetrahydrocannabinol, and carbon monoxide cross the placenta easily and may have a depressant effect on the fetal central nervous system. Only infrequent case reports have revealed any malformations, and no specific teratogenic patterns have emerged. Chromosomal damage is unlikely and of undetermined significance. Therapeutic abortion for inadvertent use of marijuana or other "street" drugs (cocaine, "angel dust," LSD, heroin, Talwin) during early pregnancy is not recommended for medical reasons alone.

Antiemetics

In June 1983, the manufacturer of Bendectin reluctantly decided to cease the production of this antiemetic. Despite no associations being found with adverse fetal effects, significant damaging publicity undermined patient confidence. If the patient is unresponsive to conservative therapy, such as frequent, small, dry meals, phenothiazine medications have been prescribed. Products such as promethazine (Phenergan) and prochlorperazine (Compazine) are not associated with an increased risk of fetal anomalies. Phenothiazines may cause drowsiness, disorientation, hypotension, and extrapyramidal signs and are not presently approved by the Food and Drug Administration for routine use during pregnancy.

Diet Pills

Many women take diet pills unintentionally at the time of conception and during early pregnancy. Appetite suppressants contain either amphetamines or phenylpropanolamine. Their chemical structure is similar to epinephrine, and the drugs exert their anorectic effects on the central and autonomic nervous systems. Although amphetamines have been suspected of having a low teratogenic potential in humans, present evidence is inconclusive and no specific anomalies have been found. The few studies involving phenmetrazine and phenylpropranolamine have not shown any causal relation between these drugs and any anomalies. Pregnancy termination is therefore not recommended under these circumstances.

Caffeine

Caffeine is present in coffee, tea, chocolate, and cola beverages, as well as in such over-the-counter medicines as headache tablets, diet pills, and cold or allergy capsules. Caffeine and its metabolites cross the placenta without apparent difficulty and are detected within the serum and urine of newborn infants. Caffeine also crosses into the breast milk, and withdrawal of moderate or continual doses may explain any jitteriness, wakefulness, or irritability in the sensitive infant.

Documentation is lacking about human malformations attributable to caffeine ingestion in normally consumed amounts. Preliminary data have suggested an association between excess caffeine intake (800 mg or more each day; six or more 6-ounce cups of coffee) and increased fetal loss. Large, well-controlled epidemiologic studies have failed to show any obvious effects from excess caffeine on the developing fetus, however. Decaffeinated beverages may be substituted, although this is not absolutely necessary.

Oral Contraceptives

When taken during early pregnancy, oral contraceptives may increase maternal nausea and vomiting and promote cholestatic jaundice. A review of the literature shows that most studies have failed to reveal an increased incidence of congenital anomalies, spontaneous abortion, and chromosomal abnormalities in pregnancies delivering at term.

A combination of anomalies involving the vertebrae, anus, cardia, trachea, esophagus, and limbs ("VACTERL" syndrome) has been associated with in-utero sex steroid exposure during early gestation. Unintentional use of sex steroids may also be associated with a slight increase in congenital limb reduction deformities or nonspecific heart defects; on the other hand, several reports have failed to confirm this cardiac teratogenicity. Masculinization of the female fetus is theoretically possible from prolonged exposure to androgen-like progestins. However, this finding has been reported in only 0.3% of all exposed female fetuses.

In our experience, the patient will discontinue oral contraceptive use soon after discovering the pregnancy. An abortion is to be discouraged, and the patient should be reassured that the risk of a malformation is no greater than the usual 2-4% incidence.

Cigarette Smoking

Of the 4,000 compounds identified in tobacco smoke, the two most studied substances are nicotine and carbon monoxide. Higher incidences of low birth weight infants, placenta previa and abruption, premature rupture of the membranes, and perinatal mortality have been reported in pregnant women who smoke. A lower mean birth weight of 100-500 gm for infants born to smokers has been the only finding reported consistently.

Nicotine can cause vasoconstriction, tachycardia, and elevated blood pressure recordings in the mother and apnea and other respiratory abnormalities in the fetus. The breast milk of heavy smokers may contain a significant amount of nicotine. Like nicotine, carbon monoxide will cross the placenta readily. Its toxicity probably relates to an impairment in tissue oxygenation by competing with oxygen for hemoglobin binding. Thus, the fetus of a smoking mother may be in a chronic state of hypoxia, which may lead to less gain in fetal weight and development.

Although there does not seem to be an increase in congenital anomalies, conflicting reports reveal a possible increased incidence of spontaneous abortion. The effect of smoking on the mental function of surviving children has not been thoroughly investigated. Along with routine questioning about smoking during the antepartum period, we counsel the patient to discontinue or at least minimize the amount of smoking. Passive exposure to smoke-filled rooms should also be avoided, although any harm to the mother or fetus is unlikely with limited exposure.

Alcohol

Teratogenic effects from alcohol have been suspected for decades, but it was not until Jones and Smith's publication in 1973 that a constellation of abnormalities was described as the "fetal alcohol syndrome." Nearly all infants were born to daily heavy alcohol drinkers.

Studies show that a daily intake of greater than 2.2 gm of ethyl alcohol per kilogram (5 ounces or six hard drinks) significantly increases the frequency of all abnormalities associated with the syndrome. Widespread effects include central nervous system dysfunction, growth deficiencies, and facial abnormalities. Mental retardation is a common manifestation. Microcephaly, hydrocephaly, and incomplete development of the cerebral cortex have also been described. Although the fetal alcohol syndrome is well established, it is uncertain whether heavy alcohol use affects early fetal loss.

No absolute safe level of consumption has been determined, so all pregnant women should be cautioned to reduce alcohol consumption to the barest minimum and encouraged to eat properly. It is unknown whether light or moderate drinking causes any added risk of malformation or abortion. Concentrations in breast milk are not significant with moderate consumption, but infant lethargy and prolonged sleeping may occur when the mother consumes excessive amounts.

Nutritional Supplements

Nutritional factors have been implicated in the etiology of hypertensive disease in pregnancy. The role of calcium in the development of hypertension has been proposed in recent epidemiologic and experimental data. Preliminary evidence of the effect of a large daily dose of calcium (2 gm) in normal pregnant women reveals a significantly lower diastolic blood pressure in the third trimester. This pattern is in contrast to that seen in similar patients who received either no treatment or a 1-gm daily dose and was seen despite no changes in blood levels of calcium, magnesium, phosphorus, and proteins.

Prenatal fluoride supplements (1 mg daily) have been recommended recently for pregnant women. Preliminary evidence suggests that enamel of teeth exposed prenatally to fluoride is resistant to caries. This is especially true of the surface enamel observed on electron microscopy.

Aspartame, a synthetic sweetener found in diet drinks, contains phenylalanine and aspartic acid. There should not be concern with its use during pregnancy. Another sweetener, saccharin, also is not associated with an increased risk of malformations.

Acne Preparations

Acne is a common dermatologic problem during pregnancy. Most acne products are topical preparations that contain benzoyl peroxide colloidal sulfur, salicylic acid, or antibiotics. In all probability, these creams, liquids, or gels are absorbed in minimal amounts and cause no harm to the fetus.

Treatment of recalcitrant cystic acne has involved cis-retinoic acid (vitamin A). Oral isotretinoin (Accutane), which contains cis-retinoic acid, is contraindicated during pregnancy because of teratogenicity in rats and rabbits. Recent case reports of major CNS defects in human fetuses and newborns have included microcephaly, hydrocephalus, and abnormalities of the external ear (micropinna, small or absent external auditory canals).

Summary

The use of any drugs during pregnancy must be sought periodically and recorded on the prenatal record. In most circumstances, the patient should be reassured that the risk to the fetus of a drug taken infrequently or inadvertently is likely negligible or miminal. No drug can be considered absolutely safe during pregnancy, because of our inability to predict the amount of drug or its metabolites being exposed to the developing embryo or fetus. A review of the current literature about the specific drug is necessary for proper counseling. Reported effects of specific drugs on the human fetus are found in Appendix A.2.

Maternal Serum Alpha-Fetoprotein (AFP) Determination

Alpha-fetoprotein (AFP) is a fetal-specific alpha-globuin that is synthesized within the fetal yolk sac, gastrointestinal tract, and liver. During the first half of pregnancy, the concentration of AFP is 100 times greater in the fetal serum than in the amniotic fluid (Fig. 1.1). Fetal and amniotic fluid concentrations peak at 14 weeks and then decline significantly until term. Maternal serum values are

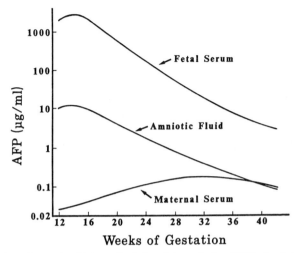

Figure 1.1. Concentrations of alpha-fetoprotein (AFP) in fetal serum, amniotic fluid, and maternal serum. (From Seppala, Amniotic Fluid, 2nd ed, New York, Excerpta Medica, 1978.)

The major clinical application of AFP testing is for the detection of fetal open neural tube defects (prevalence in U.S.A. 1-2/1000 births). Couples with an affected first degree relative should be offered an ultrasound-directed amniocentesis for the evaluation of amniotic fluid AFP. However, this approach will detect only approximately 10% of all affected infants with neural tube defects.

Recently, it has become routine for most American obstetricians to offer maternal serum AFP screening to gravidas with a negative family history. It is important that the patient understand that such screening is voluntary, and that further testing may be required if abnormal screening results occur. Routine screening on a select patient population at risk for neural tube defects or malformations is appropriate. Pregnant patients who would benefit from MSAFP determination and ultrasound exam include women with poor obstetric histories, diabetes (either by controlled diet alone or insulin dependent), a distant family member who has an open neural tube defect, or a seizure disorder and those taking valproic acid.

An initial maternal serum AFP sample is obtained at 14-18 weeks. A normal value, 0.5-2.0 multiples of the mean, rules out an open neural tube defect with about a 90% probability. Between 3-7% of American women's initial AFP will be elevated. If the value is >2.0, but <3.0 multiples of the mean (MOM) and the gestational age less than 18 weeks, a repeat sample should be obtained. Approximately half of the repeat values will be normal, and in these cases no further testing is required. The remaining patients and those gravidas whose initial maternal serum AFP is more than 3.0 MOM or whose gestational age is more than 18 weeks should be managed according to the protocol outlined in Figure 1.2.

This protocol has recently been adopted by most genetic centers because of its greater cost efficiency in patients with elevated values and more advanced gestational ages. Causes of falsely elevated maternal serum AFP values include more advanced gestational age, twins (values of 0.5-3.5 MOM are considered normal), threatened abortion, fetal death, maternal hepatitis, herpetic infection, and Rh disease. Acetlycholinesterase determination using gel electrophoresis is less influenced by fetal blood. Its use eliminates most false-positive amniotic fluid AFP values. The absence of acetylcholinesterase strongly suggests the absence of an open neural tube defect. Patients with elevated maternal serum AFP values in whom no genetic defect is found appear to be at approximately a 40% risk to deliver a low birth weight infant either due to intrauterine growth retardation or premature labor, so they should be followed closely for these problems.

Recently it has been recognized that patients with MSAFP 0.5 MOM are at increased risk to produce trisomic infants. The relative risk depends on the patient's age and her AFP level. Gravidas with serum AFP <0.05 would be managed according to the protocol outlined in Figure 1.2. Other causes for low AFP values include less advanced gestational age, trophoblastic disease, and fetal demise.

Antepartum Rh Immune Glubulin

The availability of Rho (D) immune globulin has provided a means to virtually eliminate fetal erythroblastosis from Rh disease. Unfortunately, thousands of new cases of Rh sensitization still occur annually in the United States. While certain cases result from omission or administration of inadequate doses of Rho (D) immune globulin at delivery, most Rh isoimmunization occurs from the omission of Rho (D) immune globulin at the time of elective or spontaneous abortion, ectopic pregnancy, amniocentesis, antepartum uterine bleeding, and fetal-maternal hemorrhage.

All Rh-negative unsensitized pregnant patients are eligible for antepartum Rho (D) immune globulin unless the father-to-be is known to be Rh negative. Indications for and dose of antepartum Rho (D) immune globulin are shown in Table 1.6. The dose is determined by gestational age and can be calculated by Kleihauer-Betke testing after the first 12 weeks.

We no longer perform D^u testing during maternal blood typing, since it is not cost effective. Only 1% of Rh-negative people are D - positive, and there is no harm in administering antepartum Ph immune globulin to a D -positive mother. If the cord blood at delivery is D -positive, D testing should be done on the mother.

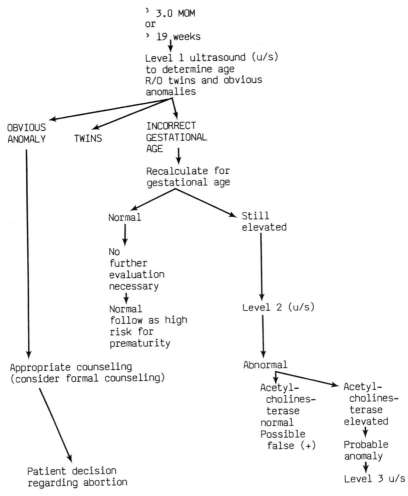

Figure 1.2. Evaluation for an elevated maternal serum AFP.

Since 1-2% of Rh-negative women will become sensitized in their current pregnancy before delivery, Rho (D) immune globulin is administerd routinely at our clinics at approximately 28 weeks to all Rh negative unsensitized patients. An indirect Coombs' test is not performed thereafter, and another injection is not given routinely for the remainder of the antepartum period.

The administration of a standard 300 mcg vial of Rh immune globulin reduces the incidence of such sensitization to 1/1000. The 300-mcg dose may cause a mildly positive Rh titer (1:4), but it is less than one-tenth of the dose required to cause significant harm to the fetus. Causes of failures of Rho (D) immune globulin include:

a) antenatal sensitization
b) inadequate dose
c) misinterpretation of maternal Rh type
d) previous Rho (D)-positive transfusion
e) failure of administration when indicated
f) immunization to cross-reacting antigen, and
g) delay in administration.

Table 1.6
Indications and Doses of Antepartum Rho (D) Immune Globulin for Rh-negative, Unsensitized Women.

Indications	Dose

Gestational age at or before 12 weeks:
    Abortion, spontaneous or induced
    Ectopic pregnancy
    Chorionic villous sampling
	50 mcg*
	    to protect against 5 ml
	    tranfused whole blood

Gestational age after 12 weeks:
    Abortion, spontaneous or induced
    Ectopic pregnancy
    Amniocentesis
    Premature labor
    Persistent vaginal bleeding
    Stillbirth
    Fetal-maternal hemorrhage
    Abdominal trauma
	300 mcg (minimum)**
	    to protect against 30 ml
	    transfused whole blood

Transfusion
    Red cells, whole blood,
        platelets or granulocytes
	300 mcg (minimum)**

*Microdose brands include MICRhoGAM and Mini-Gamulin Rh.
**Regular dose brands include RhoGAM, Gamulin Rh, and HypRho-D.

The half-life of Rho (D) immune globulin is 23 days. A repeat injection at 28 weeks and after delivery (for Rh-positive infants) is recommended for those Rh-negative women who undergo a genetic amniocentesis. This additional globulin should maintain an adequate level of antibody to prevent enhancement. If the last injection was administered 4 or more weeks previously, there is no contraindication to administering the product again.

Even though this IgG antibody will cross the placenta, it will not cause any appreciable hemolysis. There is no risk of transmission of viral diseases, including hepatitis B and AIDS, although a false-positive hepatitis serology is possible. Severe anaphylactic reaction or serum sickness is exceedingly rare. After the delivery of an Rh-positive infant, Rh immune globulin 300 mcg should be administered intramuscularly despite a weakly positive direct Coombs' titer of cord blood.

Amniocentesis before Elective Repeat Cesarean Section

Despite allowing attempts at vaginal births after cesarean section (VBAC), the majority of women choose to undergo a repeat operation. Not long ago 15-20% of admissions to the neonatal intensive care unit were the result of iatrogenic prematurity after elective induction or repeat cesarean section. The accessibility of ultrasound and amniocentesis has provided a means to determine gestational age accurately and to document pulmonary maturity. Given the current level of obstetric technology, iatrogenic prematurity after an elective delivery should be rare.

The need for accurate gestational dating cannot be overemphasized. The following factors are necesary to define a reliable gestational age:

a) The patient is initially seen during the first half of pregnancy.
b) The date of her last menses is accurately known.
c) Uterine size is consistent with gestational age between the 18th-30th gestational weeks.
d) An ultrasonic exam for gestational dating is performed before the 26th week.

Inaccurate Gestation Dating

An amniocentesis for fetal lung maturity testing should be performed when estimation of gestational age appears inaccurate. The amniocentesis should be undertaken between the presumed 37th and 38th completed weeks for nonemergent conditions. All amniocenteses should be preceded by or performed during real-time ultrasonographic visualization. Any "bloody tap" or transplacental insertion of the needle requires a nonstress test and the administration of Rh immune globulin to any Rh negative, unsensitized patients.

An amniocentesis does not need to be performed if the procedure appears to be technically difficult because of reduced amniotic fluid volume, a biparietal diameter measurement of more than 92 mm a grade 3 placenta, or free floating particulate matter in the amniotic fluid is strongly suggestive of fetal lung maturity. If concern remains about the accuracy of dating, ultrasound findings, and technical difficulties with an amniocentesis, a safe alternative is to wait to perform the surgery once labor begins.

Accurate Gestation Dating

With accurate dating or once fetal lung tests indicate maturity, an elective repeat cesarean section is performed between the 38th and 39th gestational weeks, before the onset of labor. If estimation of gestational age is accurate, an amniocentesis is not routinely recommended. Confirmation of the ultrasonic findings described above is also reassuring. Advantages to not routinely performing an amniocentesis include cost considerations and avoiding an invasive procedure.

Suggested Readings

Gestational Age Determination

Hertz RH, Sokol RJ, Knoke JD, et al: Clinical estimation of gestational age: Rules for avoiding preterm delivery. Am. J. Obstet. Gynecol. 131:395, 1978.

Cartwright PS, Victory DF, MT (ASCP), Wong SW, et al: Evaluation of the new generation of urinary pregnancy tests. Am. J. Obstet. Gynecol. 153:730-1, 1985.

Weiner CP, Sabbagha RE, Vaisrub N, et al: Ultrasonic Fetal Weight Prediction: Role of Head Circumference and Femur Length. Obstet. Gynecol. 65:812, 1985.

Warsof SL, Wolf P, Coulehan J, et al: Comparison of fetal weight estimation formulas with and without head measurements. Obstet. Gynecol. 67:569, 1986.

Hadlock FP, Harrist RB, Shah YP, et al: Estimating fetal age using multiple parameters: A prospective evaluation in a racially mixed population. Am. J. Obstet. Gynecol. 156:955-7, 1987.

Herbert WNP, Bruninghaud HM, Barefoot AB, et al: Clinical aspects of fetal heart auscultation. Obstet. Gynecol. 69:574, 1987.

Recommendations to Patients

McLaughlin C: The Black Parents Handbook: A Guide to Healthy Pregnancy, Birth, and Childcare. New York, Harcourt, Brace, Jovanovich, 1976.

Ewy D, Ewy R: Preparation for Childbirth: A Lamaze Guide. Boulder, CO, Pruett, 1976.

Nilsson L: A Child is Born. New York, Dell, 1977.

Samuels J: The Well Baby Book. New York, Summit, 1978.

Whelan E: The Pregnancy Experience: Psychology of Expectant Parenthood. New York, W.W. Norton, 1978.

Rabowitz E, Rubin G: Living with Your New Baby: A Postpartum Guide for Mothers and Fathers. New York, Franklin Walls, 1978.

Bing E: Having a Baby after 40. New York, Bantam Books, 1980.

Gresh S: Becoming a Father: A Handbook for Expectant Fathers. New York, Butterick, 1980.

The Womanly Art of Breastfeeding. Franklin Park, IL, LaLeche League International, 1981.

Acevedo ZO: The Father Book: Pregnancy and Beyond. Washington, D.C., Acropolis Books, 1981.

Mossman K, Hill L: Radiation risks in pregnancy. Obstet. Gynecol. 60:237, 1982.

Russell K: Eastman's Expectant Motherhood. Boston, Little, Brown and Co, 1983.

Automobile passenger restraints for children and pregnant women. ACOG Tech. Bull. 74, March 1983.

Lotgering F, Gilbert R, Longo L: The interactions of exercise and pregnancy: A review. Am. J. Obstet. Gynecol. 149:560, 1984.

Exercise during pregnancy and the postnatal period. ACOG Tech. Bull. May, 1985.

Chamberlain G: Effect of work during pregnancy.   Obstet. Gynecol. 65:747, 1985.

Collings C, Curet LB: Fetal heart rate response to maternal exercise. Am. J. Obstet. Gynecol. 151:498-501, 1985.

Garbaciak JA, Richter M, Miller S, et al: Maternal weight and pregnancy complications. Am. J. Obstet. Gynecol. 152:238-45, 1985.

Tierson F, Olsen C, Hook E: Nausea and vomiting of pregnancy and association with pregnancy outcome. Am. J. Obstet. Gynecol. 155:1017, 1986.

Hansen J: Older maternal age and pregnancy outcome: A review of the literature. Obstet. Gynecol. Surv. 41:726, 1986.

Rayburn W, Engdahl-Hoffman K: Gestational nausea: A role for antiemetics? Contemp. Ob/Gyn: Sept 1986, p 163.

Chapman M, Jones M, Spring J, et al: The use of a birthroom: A randomized controlled trial comparing delivery with that in a labour ward. Br. J. Obstet. Gynaecol. 93:182, 1986.

Taffel SM, Keppell KG: Advicde about weight gain during pregnancy and actual weight gain. Am. J. Public Health 76:1396, 1986.

Zuckerman BS, Frank DA, Hingson R, et al: Impact of maternal work outside the home during pregnancy on neonatal outcome. Pediatrics 77:459, 1986.

Huch R, Baumann H, Fallenstein F, et al: Physiologic changes in pregnant women and their fetuses during jet air travel. Am. J. Obstet. Gynecol. 154:996-1000, 1986.

Mehta L, Yound I: Recurrence risks for common complications of pregnancy - A review. Obstet. Gynecol. Surv. 42:128, 1987.

Poland ML, Ager JW, Olson JM: Barriers to receiving adequate prenatal care. Am. J. Obstet. Gynecol. 157:297-303, 1987.

Jarnfelt-Samsioe A: Nausea and vomiting in pregnancy: A review. Obstet. & Gynecol. Survey 41:422, 1987.

Mehta L, Young ID: Recurrence risks for common complications of pregnancy - A review. Obstet. & Gynecol. Survey 42:218, 1987.

Drug Effects on the Fetus

Briggs GG, Freeman RK, Yaffe SJ: Drugs in Pregnancy and Lactation: A
Reference Guide to Fetal and Neonatal Risk. (2nd ed). Baltimore,
Williams & Wilkins, 1986.

Rayburn WF, Zuspan FP (eds): Drug Therapy in Obstetrics and
Gynecology. (2nd ed). Norwalk, CT, Appleton-Century-Crofts, 1986.

Shepard TH: Catalog of Teratogenic Agents (5th ed).   Baltimore,
Johns Hopkins, 1986.

Hatch EE, Bracken MB: Effect of marijuana use in pregnancy on fetal
growth. Em. J. Epidemiol. 124:986, 1986.

Rubin PC: Prescribing in pregnancy. Br. Med. J. 293:1415, 1986.

Koren G, Edwards MB, Miskin M: Antenatal sonography of fetal
malformations associated with drugs and chemicals: A guide.   Am. J.
Obstet. Gynecol. 156:79, 1987.

Piper JM, Baum C, Kennedy DL: Prescription drug use before and during
pregnancy in a Medicaid population. Am. J. Obstet. Gynecol. 157:148,
1987.

Maternal Serum Alpha-Fetoprotein Determination

Milunsky A, Alpert E: Results and benefits of a maternal serum alpha-
fetoprotein screening program. JAMA 252:1438, 1984.

Davis RO, Cosper P, Huddleston JF, et al: Decreased levels of amniotic
fluid alpha-fetoprotein associated with Down syndrome. Am. J. Obstet.
Gynecol. 153:541, 1985.

Hamilton MPR, Abdalla HI, Whitfield CR: Significance of raised
maternal serum alpha-fetoprotein in singleton pregnancies with normally
formed fetuses. Obstet. Gynecol. 65:465, 1985.

Doran TA, Cadesky K, Wong PY, et al: Maternal serum alpha-fetoprotein
and fetal autosomal trisomies. Am. J. Obstet Gynecol. 154:277, 1986.

Simpson JL, Baum LD, Depp R, et al: Low maternal serum alpha-
fetoprotein and perinatal outcome. Am. J. Obstet. Gynecol. 156:852,
1987.

Nelson LH, Bensen J, Burton BK: Outcomes in patients with unusually high maternal serum alpha-fetoprotein levels. Am. J. Obstet. Gynecol. 157:572, 1987.

DiMaio MS, Baumgarten A, Greenstein RM, et al: Screening for fetal Down's syndrome in pregnancy by measuring maternal serum alpha-fetoprotein levels. N. Engl. J. Med. 317:342, 1987.

Antepartum Rh Immune Globulin

The selective use of Rho (D) immune globulin (RhIG). ACOG Tech. Bull. 61, March, 1981.

Adams MM, Marks JS, Kaplan JP: Cost implications of routine antenatal administration of Rh immune globulin. Am. J. Obstet. Gynecol. 149:633, 1984.

Nusbacher V, Nichols E: Routine antepartum Rh immune globulin administration. JAMA 252:2763, 1984.

Prevention of Rho(D) isoimmunization. ACOG Tech. Bull. 79, August, 1984.

Bowman JM: Controversies in Rh prophyllaxis: Who needs Rh immune globulin and when should it be given? Am. J. Obstet. Gynecol. 151:289, 1985.

Kennedy MS: Rho(D) immune globulin. In Rayburn W, Zuspan F (eds): Drug Therapy in Obstetrics and Gynecology. E. Norwalk, CT, Appleton-Century-Crofts, 1986, pp 233-240.

Amniocentesis before Elective Repeat Cesarean Section

Frigoletto FD, Phillippe M, Davies IJ, et al.: Avoiding iatrogenic prematurity with elective repeat cesarean section without the routine use of amniocentesis. Am. J. Obstet. Gynecol. 137:521, 1980.

Hayashi RH, Berry JL, Castillo MS: Use of ultrasound biparietal diameter in timing of repeat cesarean section. Obstet. Gynecol. 57:325, 1981.

Chervenak FA, Shamsi H: Is amniocentesis necessary before elective repeat cesarean section? Obstet. Gynecol. 60:305, 1982.

Golde, SH, Petrucha R, Meade KW, et al.: Fetal lung maturity: The adjunctive use of ultrasound. Am. J. Obstet. Gynecol. 142:445, 1982.

Read J: The scheduling of repeat cesarean section operations: Prospective management protocol experience. Am. J. Obstet. Gynecol. 151:557, 63, 1985.

Chapter 2

Medical Disorders During Pregnancy

Gestational Diabetes

A woman is more likely to develop glucose intolerance during pregnancy because of counterinsulin hormones and enzymes produced primarily by the placenta. One to six percent of all women in the United States will have documented glucose intolerance during pregnancy. When glucose intolerance is diagnosed, the following conditions are more common: fetal loss (up to 2-3 times greater than the general population), fetal macrosomia and its attendant complications (even when fasting glucose concentrations are normal), deterioration of glucose metabolism resulting in the need for insulin (in approximately 20% of gestational diabetics), increased risk of operative or mechanical deliveries because of increased fetal size, and overt diabetes being developed later (within 20 years in 20% of gestational diabetics).

In the past, obstetricians tended to selectively screen for gestational diabetes when various historical or clinical risk factors were present. Several recent studies have indicated that the incidence of gestational diabetes is the same whether or not risk factors are present. Therefore, the National Institute of Health, American Diabetes Association, and American College of Obstetricians and Gynecologists recommend that all pregnant patients be screened for diabetes, regardless of whether they were screened in a prior pregnancy.

Diagnosis

Screening for gestational diabetes involves obtaining a serum glucose determination 1-hr after a 50-gm glucose challenge. This is preferred over the 2-hr, 100-gm glucola test, since there is less patient nausea and less waiting time. The test is also less expensive than the more cumbersome 3-hr glucose tolerance test (GTT). A 1-hr serum value of 140 mg/dl requires more definitive evaluation by a 3-hr GTT. Capillary (fingerstick) whole blood glucose determinations can be performed with a reflectance meter and values are slightly higher than corresponding plasma or serum levels. A 1-hr whole blood glucose of 170 mg/dl suggests the need for a 3-hr GTT.

A 3-hr GTT using a 100-gm glucose load requires fasting blood as well as a sampling at 1-, 2-, and 3-hr intervals. Criteria for GTT interpretation are shown in Table 2.1. Any two values greater than the expected levels are diagnostic of gestational onset glucose intolerance (Class A diabetes).

Table 2.1
Detection of Diabetes in Pregnancy

Test	Time (hr)	Plasma Glucose *(mg/dl)	Capillary Glucose *(mg/dl)
Screening 50 gm oral glucose No preparation Without regard to time of last meal or time of day	1	140*	170
Oral glucose tolerance+ 100 gm oral glucose			
Overnight fast for 8-14 hours	Fasting 1	105 190	115 210
At least 3 days of un- restricted diet with more than 150 g carbohydrate Patient at rest during study	2 3	165 145	185 155

*Upper limit of normal
+Diagnosis of gestational diabetes is made when any two values are exceeded.

Management

Adequate control of the mother's glucose levels by dietary manipulation and blood glucose monitoring is necessary to decrease the increased risk of perinatal morbidity, primarily from fetal macrosomia and its attendant medical and metabolic complications. Most patients will be treated sufficiently with a daily diet consisting of 30-35 cal/kg ideal body weight. Approximately 40-50% of caloric intake should be foods containing complex carbohydrates. One hundred grams of protein are also essential each day. Sweets, "junk" food, and greasy fried foods should be avoided.

More frequent clinic visits are recommended (every two weeks until 36 weeks, then weekly thereafter) and glucose monitoring should be performed periodically. Fasting and 2-hr postprandial glucose determinations are recommended during the more frequent examinations. The patient should be instructed to avoid eating after midnight, have her "fasting" blood drawn when seen initially in the clinic, then eat a "regular" meal at the cafeteria or brought from home before returning in 2 hr for a postprandial glucose determination. A fasting serum glucose level less than 105 mg/dl and a 2-hr postprandial value less than 120 mg/dl are desired. Capillary blood glucose determinations using a reflectance photometer may be more convenient and cost effective in the clinic setting. These values tend to be slightly higher than plasma levels. Therefore, a fasting capillary glucose level of less than 115 mg/dl and two hour postprandial less than 140 mg/dl are desirable.

If either glucose value exceeds recommended levels, it is necessary to get a more detailed history of the patient's diet, consult a dietitian, and consider insulin therapy. Any patient with persistently elevated blood glucose requires further evaluation in the hospital, probably with the administration of insulin. To decrease the risk of fetal macrosomia, certain class A diabetics may be started on 10-20 units of intermediate acting purified or synthetic insulin each morning, preferably before the 28th week. Under these circumstances, more frequent 2-hr postprandial glucose determinations using a portable reflectance meter must be obtained at home or during the weekly examinations.

Gestational age should be determined accurately. Ultrasound is quite helpful and may also be used during the last 2 months of pregnancy to search for signs of a large-for-gestational age fetus or polyhydramnios.

Pregnancies of class A diabetic patients may be described as being either complicated (co-existent hypertension or history of previous stillbirth) or uncomplicated (all others). Uncomplicated Class A patients are at low risk for antepartum stillbirth and may be followed until labor occurs spontaneously.

The need for antepartum fetal testing among uncomplicated Class A patients is not firmly established. Fetal movement charting often provides a useful method for monitoring and is recommended beginning at approximately the 34th gestational week. Many authorities advocate nonstress testing beginning at approximately the 36th gestational week. Complicated Class A pregnancies are at increased risk for antepartum stillbirth, so fetal movement charting and nonstress testing should be initiated at 32 weeks gestation or earlier depending on the patient's previous obstetrical history. Gestation should not be allowed to advance beyond the estimated date of confinement regardless of whether or not there is a complication.

Fetal pulmonary maturity is frequently delayed in Class A patients, so an amniocentesis for pulmonary maturity testing should usually be performed before most elective deliveries. The physician who will care for the infant should also be notified well before the anticipated delivery because there is a significantly greater risk of neonatal complications even in well-controlled Class A diabetics. Some women with low mean glucose values may still deliver macrosomic infants.

Insulin-Dependent Diabetes

Fifty years ago, maternal mortality among insulin-requiring diabetics was 50% and perinatal mortality was nearly 100%. Maternal mortality is now rare, and perinatal mortality is related to a certain extent to the duration of maternal diabetes and any evidence of vascular disease. Current management techniques have made perinatal survival less dependent on diabetes class. Except for Class H patients, perinatal mortality is less than 5% in most tertiary centers. These improvements have resulted from the meticulous execution of comprehensive protocols for the management of pregnant diabetics. Table 2.2 lists the current classification of diabetes during pregnancy.

Table 2.2
Classification of Diabetics during Pregnancy

Class	Description
A	Gestational onset diabetes, adequate control by diet alone
B	Overt diabetes, onset after age 20 or duration 10 yr or less
C	Overt diabetes, onset at age 10-19 or duration 10-19 yr
D	Overt diabetes, duration more than 20 yr or onset before age 10, or benign retinopathy
F	Nephropathy (proteinuria, azotemia)
R	Proliferative retinopathy (retinitis proliferans)
H	Arteriosclerotic heart disease
I	Renal transplant

Because of the factors enumerated in the preceding section, maternal glucose control is often difficult during pregnancy. Hypoglycemia is common in the first and third trimesters, while hyperglycemic tendencies are frequent in the second and third trimesters. Ketoacidosis occurs in pregnant patients at elevated glucose levels much lower than in non-pregnant patients. Urinary tract and surgical infections are also common. Hypertensive disorders occur relatively frequently in the more advanced classes. Cesarean section rates are high, often being 50% at most tertiary centers. Progression of proliferative retinopathy occurs in 30-50% of Class R patients.

Although the etiology of antepartum stillbirth in diabetic pregnancy is not firmly established, the application of various antepartum fetal testing modalities has decreased the stillbirth rate. Fifty to seventy percent of perinatal deaths result from congenital anomalies which are found in approximately 6-8% of diabetic pregnancies. Because increased placental transfer of glucose, amino acids, and free fatty acids results in fetal hyperinsulinemia, adipose deposition is promoted and infants of diabetic mothers experience higher rates of macrosomia and attendant birth trauma. Neonatal hypoglycemia and hypocalcemia are common. Lung maturation is delayed in some infants causing hyaline membrane disease and transient tachypnea to be more common than in those delivered to mothers without diabetes.

Cautious glucose control appears to reduce the incidence of maternal complications. Recent evidence also suggests that normoglycemia at conception and in the first trimester may decrease the incidence of congenital abnormalities and spontaneous abortions. Some authorities believe that normoglycemia in the latter portion of pregnancy may reduce the incidence of nenonatal complications. While the relationship between neonatal complications and maternal glucose control is not firmly established, all investigators believe that attempts should be made to achieve the best possible control.

Clinic Visits and Hospitalizations

At the initial prenatal visit, we find that many patients with insulin-dependent diabetes, regardless of the duration or age at onset, require hospitalization for control of blood glucose, patient education, baseline renal function tests, EKG, and ophthalmologic examination. Hospitalization may be avoided if patient knowledge about pregnancy expectations is adequate and glucose control is already strict. If there is evidence for renal, retinal, or cardiovascular compromise, the possibility of pregnancy termination in the first 15 weeks of pregnancy should be discussed.

Once discharged, the patient should visit the clinic every 1 or 2 weeks, depending on the compliance in home blood glucose monitoring and the level of her control. Beyond the 30th week, the patient should be seen in the clinic on a weekly basis, and hospitalization is necessary for inadequate glucose control or any worrisome obstetric or other medical complication.

Control of Serum Glucose

A fair correlation exists between mean daily capillary glucose values over 4 weeks and the subsequent glycosylated hemoglobin (Hb A_{1c}) level. We recommend that a Hgb A value should be determined under the following circumstances: 1) initial visit, 2) when there is a question of inadequate control, 3) when seen initially after maternal transport, or 4) after delivery of a large-for-gestational age infant. A markedly elevated Hb A_{1c} before 14 weeks gestation is associated with a 22% incidence of major congenital malformations compared with 5% or less if the value is within the normal range. A maternal serum alpha-fetoprotein value should be determined between 16-18 weeks.

To avoid ketosis and to decrease the risk of perinatal mortality, strict control of glucose levels is desirable by adjustments of insulin dose and redistribution of caloric intake. Most patients can learn how to determine and record blood sugar results in a cost effective manner at home using a reflectance meter (Accucheck, Dextrometer, Glucometer), either loaned from the clinic or purchased (approximately $100-$200). We recommend that blood sugar determinations be made four times daily (usually 7:00 a.m., 11:00 a.m., 4:00 p.m., 10:00 p.m.).

Ideally, a fasting capillary glucose should be less than 115 mg/dl, a 2-hr postprandial glucose determination less than 140 mg/dl, and before meals less than 110 mg/dl. Glucose determinations may be every other day rather than daily during the first half of pregnancy if control is adequate and no insulin reactions have occurred.

Control of glucose levels should ideally be as strict as possible. We classify glucose control in the following manner: strict if preprandial glucose values average 100 mg/dl or less, fair if 101 to 149 mg/dl, and poor if 150 mg/dl or more.

The patient's diet should be the same as that described for the Class A diabetic. In addition, a readjustment of caloric intake throughout the day may be necessary to more adequately control the blood sugars.

Insulin should be NPH (long acting) and regular (short acting) mixed together, and most patients require dosages in the morning and evening. Morning doses are often a mixture of NPH and regular insulin in a 2:1 ratio; the evening dose, usually one half the morning dose, is a 1:1 combination of NPH and regular insulin. A third dose of regular insulin at noon or before bedtime is occasionally necessary. Portable or implantable intravenous or subcutaneous insulin pumps have been used when strict or fair glucose control has not been achievable.

Purified pork insulin or recombinant DNA insulin (Humalin) may lower insulin requirements, decrease lipohypertrophy, and lessen insulin antibody formation and placental transfer in comparison with less pure preparations. The former should be prescribed to all new insulin-dependent diabetics and may be helpful when difficulty is encountered in establishing adequate glucose control.

Frequent episodes of hypoglycemia (less than 60 mg/dl) or hyperglycemia (greater than 200 mg/dl) should be avoided, even though no relation exists between maternal hypoglycemia and damage to the fetus. Although rarely necessary, the patient's family should be instructed on the use and administration of intramuscular glucagon (using 1 mg kits) and buccal glucose tablets to treat a hypoglycemia reaction which occurs most often at night. We have been recommending a 0.5 mg dose of glucagon, then the ingestion of juice, rather than administering a full dose to minimize any profound adrenergic response. Ketonuria is seen occasionally in fasting states (early morning clinic) but is not necessarily worrisome if serum glucose levels are appropriate and ketonuria is absent later in the day.

Diabetic ketoacidosis is associated with intrauterine fetal demise. However, it is uncommonly seen in pregnancies in which glucose is strictly monitored. Fluid and metabolic derangements should be corrected as soon as possible by frequent evaluation of the clinical and laboratory status. Baseline serum glucose, ketone, potassium, sodium, BUN, creatinine, and HCO_3 levels should be determined. Bicarbonate therapy (1 ampule, 44 meq) is to be started in the presence of a pH less than 7.1, shock, or coma. A bolus of regular insulin at 0.15 units/kg body weight should be followed by a constant insulin infusion at 0.15 units/kg body weight/hr (5-10 units are mixed with 100 ml of normal saline). The maintenance dose may be doubled if the serum glucose value has not fallen to 200 mg/dl during the first 2 hours. A 5% glucose solution should be used once the glucose concentration falls to 250 mg/dl. The intravenous infusion may be discontinued once the pH becomes normal. A sliding scale insulin regimen should be continued until a liquid diet is tolerated. Long-acting insulin may be added the next morning.

Fetal Well-Being Tests

Maternal serum alpha-fetoprotein (AFP) levels should be drawn between the 15th and 20th weeks to screen for any elevation from open neural tube defects. Ultrasound for fetal age and growth assessments should be done on the initial visit and at 4-6 week intervals.

The risk of intrauterine fetal demise increases as gestation proceeds beyond 30 weeks. The etiology of fetal death is often unclear; however, patients with preeclampsia, uteroplacental vascular lesions, and maternal hyperglycemia are at increased risk. The patient should be instructed on fetal movement charting beginning at the 29th gestational week. Weekly nonstress tests, contraction stress tests or biophysical profiles should be initiated sometime between the 28th and 32nd gestational weeks and increased to twice weekly by the 34th gestational week. Testing should begin earlier and be undertaken more frequently in the presence of cardiovascular disease, poor glucose control, or poor obstetric history.

Prolonged hospitalization before delivery is no longer routine provided that excellent metabolic control and adequate fetoplacental testing can be accomplished on an outpatient basis. Pregnancy may be allowed to continue until the 38th week when most authorities recommend that an amniocentesis for fetal lung maturity testing be performed. The lung maturity screen should include a determination of the lecithin/sphingomyelin (L/S) ratio and phosphatidylglycerol (PG). An L/S ratio of 3 alone or an L/S ratio of 2-3 with a positive PG strongly suggests fetal lung maturity with a very minimal risk of subsequent development of hyaline membrane disease. Induction should be undertaken if lung maturity is present, the fetus is in a vertex presentation, the estimated fetal weight is less than 4,000 gms, and the Bishop score is favorable. If the cervix is unfavorable, it is permissible to delay delivery until the anticipated due date, provided the metabolic and fetoplacental status remains stable. If the estimated fetal weight is more than 4,000 gms or if the fetus is in a breech presentation, cesarean delivery is usually performed to prevent birth trauma.

Prolonged hospitalization may be required when there is evidence of worsening end organ damage (proliferative retinopathy, nephropathy), hypertension, inadequate glucose control, poor patient compliance, or abnormal fetoplacental function tests. Every attempt should be made to optimize glucose control. In addition to daily fetal movement charting, the frequency of fetoplacental testing should be increased. An amniocentesis may be performed before the 38th week. Delivery is usually dependent on the worsening of any of the above conditions or the presence of fetal lung maturity. Cesarean section is often necessary because the cervix remains unfavorable; however, the use of prostaglandin E_2 gel in effacing the cervix is gaining wider acceptance.

The pediatric staff must be notified in advance of any impending delivery, since these infants usually require intravenous glucose therapy and may need respiratory support. Metabolic complications include hyperbilirubinemia, hypoglycemia, hypocalcemia, and poor feeding. The reported incidence of major malformations in infants born to diabetics is 8%, and perinatal mortality (approximately half are stillbirths) at most perinatal regional centers is less than 5%.

Insulin Requirements during and after Delivery

Before Labor
Despite close antepartum glucose monitoring, maternal hypoglycemia or hyperglycemia may occur during labor and delivery and neonatal glucose control may be significantly compromised. Before the anticipated day of delivery, the usual evening dose of insulin is given. The patient is kept NPO after midnight, and insulin on the day of delivery is given intravenously. Before induction of labor or cesarean section, a serum glucose is drawn and an intravenous line is begun. A D_5W drip is run at 150 ml/hr (7.5 gm/hr).

Intrapartum
The desired goal is to maintain a serum glucose within the 60-120 mg/dl range with serum glucoses being determined every 1-3 hours depending on the degree of control. In our practices insulin is given intravenously with capillary glucose levels being determined with a bedside glucometer.

Thirty units of regular insulin are drawn into a 50 ml syringe, and mixed with 50 ml of normal saline (0.6 units insulin/ml). The insulin may adhere to the syringe, so 1 ml of the patient's blood should be drawn into the syringe and mixed well.

A constant rate pump is used to infuse the insulin at 2 ml/hr (1.2 units/hr) in a "piggy-back" manner. Insulin requirements during labor are often negligible. The average patient requires 1.2 units of insulin per hour (range 0-3 units/hr) and usually no greater than 1.5 units/hr. Oxytocin may be infused through the same vein using another line at a keep-open rate.

Postpartum

Placental hormones are metabolized and eliminated rapidly after delivery, and insulin requirements decrease dramatically. In our experience, pre-pregnancy insulin requirements are usually reached within 4-7 days after delivery, and dose requirements are approximately one-half to one-third those necessary for adequate control late in pregnancy.

If delivery was vaginal, insulin infusion should continue until the patient is transferred from the recovery area. In the first few days after delivery, strict glucose control is not necessary, and we strive for glucose values less than 200 mg/dl. Regular insulin may be administered by a sliding scale regimen based on blood glucometer results obtained every 4-6 hrs. Five units of regular insulin should be administered subcutaneously for a glucose level of 200-249 mg/dl, 10 units for a level 250-299 mg/dl, and 15 units of 300 mg/dl or higher.

After cesarean section, insulin infusion may be continued through the first day or until oral intake is tolerated, with bedside glucose monitoring every 2-4 hours. Minimal or no insulin is usually necessary. Insulin requirements do not appear to be affected greatly by the patient's mode of delivery or whether breast feeding is undertaken. NPH or Lente is usually begun around the 4th postpartum day after 1 full day of eating solid foods.

If the patient is a Class A diabetic, particulary if insulin was only required during the third trimester, insulin is usually unnecessary before discharge. Patient instructions should include an emphasis on proper nutrition, physician notification of excess fatigue, and continued glucose monitoring (fasting and postprandial two or three times weekly). A glucose tolerance test should be scheduled at the 6-week postpartum visit if glucose values have not returned to normal.

Obesity

There is disagreement about the proper definition of obesity in pregnancy, although various authors have suggested prepregnancy weights greater than 175 pounds or at least 40% (usually 100 pounds or more) above ideal body weight. Obese women are at increased risk for hypertension, gestational diabetes, urinary tract infection, and episiotomy or wound infections. Pregnancy dating is often inaccurate because of irregular menstrual cycles and difficulties with uterine height examinations.

In most studies, maternal mortality rates are increased, largely from thromboembolic, infectious, and anesthetic complications. Fetal macrosomia is also more common. Although perinatal mortality usually not increased and low birth weight infants are uncommon, an optimal pregnancy outcome is associated with a weight gain of at least 15 pounds for these mothers.

Antepartum Management

1. Nutritional counseling at first visit and follow-up visits

2. Screening urine culture
3. Ultrasound at approximately 20 weeks to confirm pregnancy dating
4. Diabetes screen initially and at 24-28 weeks (using the 1-hr, 50 gm glucose challenge)
5. Frequent blood pressure monitoring using a large cuff if arm circumference is 35 cm or more
6. Prophylactic rest at least 1 hour each day in the third trimester
7. Pulmonary function tests followed by an anesthesia consult in early third trimester should be considered if the patient is morbidly obese.

Intrapartum and Postpartum Management

1. Prophylactic heparin (5,000 units subcutaneously every 12 hrs) during labor and until fully ambulatory
2. Notify anesthesia staff of patient's presence in labor and delivery
3. Careful monitoring for pre-eclampsia using a large blood pressure cuff
4. Careful attention to the progress of labor
5. Anticipation of fetal shoulder dystocia because of possible macrosomia
6. Meticulous hemostasis during episiotomy repair
7. If cesarean section is required: a) prophylactic antibiotics, b) vertical incision with Smead-Jones closure or Pfannenstiel incision, and c) self contained suction drains (such as a Jackson Pratt drain) in subcutaneous space
8. Early ambulation
9. Continued nutritional counseling in the postpartum period

Chronic Hypertension

Approximately 2% of all pregnant patients will have chronic hypertension which is defined as any interval or sustained elevation of the blood pressure (140/90 mm Hg or greater) before pregnancy or before 20 weeks of the present pregnancy. These patients are frequently obese and may have been on diuretic therapy or a beta-blocking antihypertensive medication. A search for end organ damage such as renal or cardiac disease is necessary, since either may affect the prognosis for the mother and unborn infant.

Antepartum Management

The preliminary outpatient investigation (inpatient if elevated blood pressure) should include: a) a 24-hr urine for protein and creatinine clearance, b) serum electrolytes, c) urinalysis and urine culture, d) ultrasound examination, e) electrocardiogram, f) trial off medications if normotensive, and g) patient instruction on home blood pressure monitoring. Return clinic visits should be a minimum of every 3 weeks until 20 weeks, every 2 weeks until 32 weeks, and every week after 32 weeks. The patient should be instructed on recording blood pressures at home and sharing these results with her physician. Bedrest is encouraged for one or more hours each afternoon.

Methyldopa (Aldomet) is the drug of choice (up to 500 mg q.i.d.) because it poses minimal risk to the fetus and there has been extensive experience with its use during pregnancy. Diuretics are seldom if ever necessary and should be avoided because of fetal electrolyte imbalances, thrombocytopenia, jaundice, and even death (especially sudden large doses which deplete intravascular volume). The diuretic drugs may be continued only if the patient has well-documented hypertension and was treated with them prior to her pregnancy, or if she develops congestive heart failure. No second drug to treat hypertension during pregnancy has been clearly shown to be preferable, even though hydralazine is most commonly used. If a second drug is necessary and hydralazine is ineffective, propranolol may be used. Propranolol should be discontinued shortly before labor or delivery to minimize effects seen in the neonate (bradycardia, hypoglycemia, depressed respirations). The newer beta-blocking drugs (atenolol, labetalol) are thought to be safe using the above precautions. The safety of calcium channel-blocking drugs (nifedipine) remains unclear presently.

Fetal heart rate testing is usually begun at the 32nd-34th gestational weeks if medications are used or if the hypertension worsens. Serial ultrasound exams to assess fetal growth and placental morphology are recommended early in pregnancy and usually no more frequently than every 3 weeks. Daily fetal movement charting should begin during the early third trimester.

Hospitalization is indicated for a persistent elevation of systolic/diastolic values 30/15 mm Hg above previous levels, signs of superimposed preeclampsia, or a suspicion of fetal growth retardation or distress.

Consider delivery as soon as fetal lung maturity is attained or by 40 weeks if fetal growth has been normal and maternal blood pressure has been well controlled. If delivery is anticipated before 34 weeks, glucocorticoids may be given to enhance fetal lung maturity if the mother's condition is stable and blood pressures are no more than 160/105.

Intrapartum Management

If superimposed preeclampsia develops, intravenous magnesium sulfate should be started for seizure prophylaxis and delivery planned. Continuous electronic fetal heart rate monitoring is recommended.

Epidural anesthesia is permissible, as long as the blood pressure is not greater than 160/105 and an experienced anesthesiologist is available. Bearing-down efforts by the mother should be avoided, and low forceps delivery may be necessary to shorten the second stage of labor.

Pregnancy-Induced Hypertension

Next to anemia, hypertension is the most common medical complication during pregnancy. Pregnancy-induced hypertension is more common than chronic hypertension during pregnancy and affects up to 10% of all pregnancies. Hypertension during pregnancy is defined as any blood pressure elevation of 140/90 or greater or any elevation of the systolic/diastolic values of more than 30/15 on two occasions 6 hrs apart.

Pregnancy-induced hypertension is often fluctuant and has an onset beyond the first 20 weeks. Differentiating between pregnancy-induced hypertension and mild preeclampsia is often difficult, but preeclampsia should be suspected if there is a weight gain of 2 pounds or more per week or persistent proteinuria of greater than 300 mg but less than 5 gm/24 hr. In either circumstance, end organ damage is not usually extensive enough to cause liver dysfunction, central nervous system involvement, coagulopathies, or pulmonary edema.

Surveillance Techniques

The following measures are recommended in monitoring the mother and fetus during the third trimester. If blood pressure values remain elevated at home and in the clinic, hospitalization is necessary.

Maternal
1. Check for headaches, blurred vision, abdominal pain, chest pain, respiratory symptoms, brisk deep tendon reflexes, and clonus
2. Instruct patient on home blood pressure monitoring
3. Weigh daily
4. Urinary output daily
5. Dipstick for proteinuria daily
6. High protein diet (100 gm daily) if proteinuria
7. Salt substitute, no diuretic therapy
8. Complete blood count and peripheral blood smear (burr cells, schistocytes, polychromasia) on admission and as indicated
9. Liver function study (SGOT) on admission and as indicated
10. Coagulation study (especially platelets) on admission and as indicated
11. Renal function testing (24-hr urine for protein and creatinine clearance) on admission and as indicated.

Fetal
1. Daily fetal movement charting
2. Nonstress or contraction stress testing weekly or semi-weekly
3. Ultrasound, biophysical and fetal growth assessment every 3 weeks or sooner if concern. Consider umbilical doppler flow studies.

Therapy in Hospital

1. Bedrest in left lateral decubitus position with bathroom privileges

2. If hyperreflexia, clonus, or BP more than 150/105, begin intravenous magnesium sulfate while monitoring urine output
3. Intermittent boluses of intravenous hydralazine 5-15 mg if BP more than 160/105
4. Pregnancy intervention if evidence of fetal lung maturity, fetal distress, deteriorating maternal end organ function or worsening persistently elevated blood pressure values
5. Discharge home only if the reliable patient can remain sedentary, is asymptomatic with no laboratory abnormalities, can monitor her urine output/protein and blood pressure daily, and lives nearby so that she can be seen twice weekly in clinic. A visiting home health nurse is often helpful.

Severe Preeclampsia or Eclampsia

Severe preeclampsia or eclampsia is an extension of pregnancy-induced hypertension or mild preeclampsia. Hospitalization is required for immediate attention to the mother and fetus. Under these circumstances, there is a greater likelihood of placenta abruption, fetal distress, and fetal demise, along with end organ changes in the mother such as renal failure, liver failure, cerebrovascular accident, heart failure, consumptive coagulopathy, and thrombocytopenia. The primary goals of therapy include stabilizing the maternal blood pressure, correcting any accompanying medical complications, and delivering the fetus in the near future.

General Recommendations

1. Admit to labor floor for close monitoring
2. Strict bedrest in a lateral position and quiet environment
3. Seizure precautions (side rails up, tongue blade, oral airway)
4. Foley catheter drainage for output measurement
5. External monitoring of fetal heart rate and any spontaneous uterine activity
6. Notify pediatricians of patient's status

Surveillance Techniques (frequency dependent on clinical status)

1. Intake and output: hourly measure of urine volume, specific gravity, and quantitative protein
2. Blood pressure, respirations, pulse hourly
3. Deep tendon reflexes (patellar-depressed or brisk), clonus
4. Bedside ultrasound examination and nonstress test
5. Immediate laboratory tests:
   a. Type and screen for possible whole blood administration
   b. Complete blood count with peripheral blood smear
   c. Urinalysis
   d. Serum electrolytes, BUN, creatinine

    e. Platelets and fibrinogen
    f. SGOT
    g. 24-hr urine collection for protein and creatinine clearance determinations
6. Frequent laboratory tests:
    a. Hematocrit
    b. Serum electrolytes
    c. Platelet count
    d. 24-hr urine for creatinine clearance and protein

Therapy

1. Intravenous magnesium sulfate with a 4-6 gm loading dose and 1-3 gm/hr maintenance dose
2. Intermittent intravenous hydralazine 5-15 mg to lower blood pressure to within a 140-155/90-105 range. Persistently elevated blood pressures may be lowered using continuous intravenous hydralazine (40 mg in 500 ml D_5W), carefully titrated according to present recordings. A reduction in placental blood flow is possible with an abrupt decrease in blood pressure. Nitroprusside using an infusion pump or a calcium channel-blocker such as nifedipine should be reserved for refractory hypertensive emergencies and may be dangerous to the fetus.
3. Nasal oxygen 5-7 liters/min if eclampsia
4. Deliver once maternal condition is stable
    a. Induction of labor if cephalic presentation and cervix is favorable. Fetal monitoring and maternal observation for excess vaginal bleeding or uterine tenderness.
    b. Cesarean section if cervix unfavorable, suspected fetal distress without imminent vaginal delivery, or other obstetric conditions (twins, breech, placenta previa, infant anticipated to weigh less than 1,500 gms). Plasma expanders such as albumin or plasmanate may be used to increase a low CVP reading.
5. Same parameters to be monitored postpartum with continued intravenous magnesium sulfate for next 12-24 hrs. Intravenous hydralazine as necessary. Avoid excess intravenous sodium and fluid overload (D5 1/2 NS at less than 200 ml/hr).
6. Consider a CVP or Swan-Ganz catheter placement in the presence of renal failure, heart failure, or persistently high blood pressure recordings despite parenteral antihypertensive medications.

Cardiac Disorders

Cardiac disease is found in 0.9-3.7% of all pregnant women. Improvements in antibiotic prophylaxis for rheumatic fever and surgical correction of congenital lesions have reduced the number of childbearing women with rheumatic heart disease and increased those with corrected congenital defects. Intravascular volume, heart rate, stroke volume, and cardiac output all increase beginning early in pregnancy and reach a peak at approximately 28-30 weeks. These changes remain relatively stable and decrease slightly near term. The increases are further magnified during labor and the immediate postpartum period.

As a result of these physiologic alterations, there is a marked increase in cardiac work. Thus, the pregnant cardiac patient is subjected to significant stress in the antepartum and peripartum periods. Her prognosis depends on the functional capacity of her heart, the presence or absence of other diseases complicating the pregnancy (such as hypertension, infection, etc.), the quality of her medical care, and the resources available in her family and community.

Historical and Clinical Findings

Symptoms such as fatigue and mild dyspnea and physical findings such as a systolic murmur, third heart sound, and edema may be signs of cardiac disease in non-pregnant women but are usually normal physiological alterations during pregnancy. Further evaluation for cardiac disease is warranted if any of the following symptoms or physical findings are present: dyspnea severe enough to limit activity, progressive orthopnea, paroxysmal nocturnal dyspnea, hemoptysis, syncope immediately following activity, chest pain with an anginal pattern associated with physical activity or emotional stress, greater than a III/IV systolic murmur (diastolic, prediastolic, or continuous), unequivocal cardiac enlargement, severe arrhythmia, or cyanosis or clubbing.

The New York Heart Association Classification in Table 2.3 may be used to classify cardiac patients during pregnancy. The prognosis for the pregnancy outcome can be assessed to a certain extent using this classification. If medication is required to maintain a lower class, the prognosis is somewhat worse.

General Recommendations

The initial history and physical examination should include a baseline ECG, an echocardiogram, and a cardiology consult. In general, the treatment of most serious cardiac disorders in pregnancy should follow the same principles as in the non-pregnant patient (Table 2.4). The patient should be seen weekly or biweekly in the obstetric clinic.

Infections may predispose to cardiac failure. Patients should be instructed to report any signs of infection to their physician and to avoid individuals with respiratory infections. Antibiotic prophylaxis against rheumatic fever (a monthly injection of benzathine penicillin (Bicillin) 1,200,000 units, or penicillin G 200,000 units orally b.i.d.) should be used in all patients with well-documented rheumatic heart disease.

Table 2.3
New York Heart Association Classification

Class 1: Patients have no limitations of physical activity. Ordinary physical activity does not cause undue fatigue, palpitations, dyspnea, or anginal pain.

Class 2: Patients with slight limitation of physical activity. Ordinary physical activity results in fatigue, palpitations, dyspnea, or anginal pain.

Class 3: Patients have marked limitations of physical activity. Less than ordinary activity causes fatigue, palpitations, dyspnea, or anginal pain.

Class 4: Patients have an inability to carry on any physical activity without discomfort. Symptoms of cardiac insufficiency or angina syndrome may be present even at rest. When physical activity is undertaken discomfort increases.

Many patients are on coumadin therapy after valve replacement. This drug should be avoided during pregnancy because of its teratogenic risk and the increased incidence of fetal and neonatal deaths from hemorrhage in the later trimesters. Heparin, 5,000-8,000 units subcutaneously every 6-8 hrs as an outpatient or intravenously using an anticoagulation dose when hospitalized, should be administered instead.

For Class 1 and Class 2 patients, management is usually on an outpatient basis. Patients should rest 1 hr several times daily to reduce cardiac work and should be hospitalized for any sign of heart failure or significant arrhythmia. Admission should be considered shortly before term for those patients who are unable to rest at home. Patients should have continuous ECG monitoring during delivery if significant abnormalities are detected on the outpatient ECG or if symptoms of ischemia occur during labor.

Because of the substantially increased risk of maternal mortality, Class 4 patients should be counseled against becoming pregnant. Extensive bedrest is necessary. Patients should be admitted routinely before term for continuous rest. A Swan-Ganz catheter and continuous ECG monitoring are required during any labor and at delivery. Determination of the pulmonary capillary wedge pressure is the most useful parameter for evaluating cardiac function in pregnant individuals with severe mitral stenosis, myocarditis, and severe pre-eclampsia. Pressures at 5-12 mm Hg are usually associated with normal vascular volume and normal ventricular function. The stressed or failing heart functions optimally at higher volumes, and wedge pressures normally range from 13-17 mm Hg. Higher values (especially above 20 mm Hg) indicate ventricular overdistention and lower values of 5 mm Hg or less indicate inadequate vascular volume.

Table 2.4
Cardiac Drugs Utilized during Pregnancy

Drug	Primary Use	Loading Dose	Maintenance Dose
Digoxin	Paroxysmal supra-ventricular tachy-arrhythmia; rate control in atrial fibrillation	0.75-1.25 mg intra-venously in 0.25 mg increments at 4-6 hr intervals 1.25-2.0 mg orally in increments at 4-6 hr invervals	0.25-0.50 mg daily, orally
Digitoxin	Same as digoxin	1.0 mg intravenously or 0.7 mg-1.2 mg orally in divided doses over 24 hr	0.1 mg-0.2 mg daily, orally
Ouabain	Rapid control in severe arrhythmias similar to other cardiac glycosides	0.3-0.5 mg intrave-nously	0.1 mg intra-venously every 4 hr
Propranolol	Atrial and ventric-ular premature beats; reentrant ventricular and supraventricular tachyarrhythmia; rate control in atrial flutter and fibrillation	0.05 mg-0.15 mg/kg intravenously by slow infusion; no more than 0.15 mg/kg should be adminis-tered in a 6 hr period	40-160 mg daily in 3-4 divided doses, orally
Disopyramide	Similar to quinidine	200-300 mg orally	400-800 mg daily, divided dose
Phenytoin	Supraventricular and ventricular arrhythmia due to digitalis toxicity	100 mg intrave-nously every 5 min until arrhythmia controlled or ad-verse effects oc-cur; total dose should not exceed 1,000 mg/24 hr 1,000 mg in divided doses orally over 24 hr	500 mg orally in divided dose

Table 2.4 (Continued)

Drug	Primary Use	Loading Dose	Maintenance Dose
Verapamil	Paroxysmal supra-ventricular tachy-arrhythmia; rate control in atrial	5-10 mg over 2-3 min; intravenous dose; may be repeated in 30 min if arrhythmia	80-120 mg 3-4 times daily, orally

Cardiac failure should be treated aggressively with rest, oxygen, rotating tourniquets, digoxin (0.5 mg IV over 10 min followed by 0.25 mg IV q 2-4 hr up to 2 mg as needed), and morphine (10-15 mg IV q 2-4 hr). Significant maternal tachycardia should be treated with propanolol (0.2-0.5 mg IV q 3 min until the rate is below 110 bpm), digoxin (as above), or cardioversion (25-100 watt seconds).

The American Heart Association recommends that antibiotics be administered before a cesarean section, urethral catheterization or during a complicated vaginal delivery in pregnant patients with valvular heart disease. They are not required in most patients with heart disease for pelvic examination, dilation and curettage of the uterus, or uncomplicated vaginal delivery, however. The recommended drug regimen for bacterial endocarditis prophylaxis is shown in Table 2.5.

Table 2.5
Drug Regimen for Bacterial Endocarditis Prophylaxis

Aqueous penicillin (2 million units) or ampicillin (1 gm) IV or IM **plus** either gentamicin (1.5 mg/kg IM or IV) or streptomycin (1 gm IM) 0.5-1 hr before the procedure

If gentamicin is used, repeat the dose of penicillin or ampicillin and gentamicin every 8 hrs for 2 additional doses

If streptomycin is used, give penicillin or ampicillin with streptomycin every 12 hrs for 2 additional doses after the procedure

If the patient is allergic to penicillin, vancomycin (1 gm IV infused over 30 min) about 1 hr before the procedure, and gentamicin or streptomycin as above can be used. The same dose of these agents may be repeated in 8-12 hrs for 2 more doses.

Beta-agonists for the treatment of premature labor are contraindicated in patients with significant cardiac disease.

Magnesium sulfate may be used cautiously, since cardiotoxicity is possible with high doses.

A cesarean section should be performed only for the usual obstetric indications. Cardiac surgery such as a commissurotomy may be performed during pregnancy but should be reserved for those patients unresponsive to medical management and preferably during the second trimester. Adequate oxygenation and mild hypothermia are desired during the procedure. Electronic fetal monitoring may be helpful since the heart rate is influenced by the maternal blood pressure and oxygenation.

Mitral Stenosis

Because the physiologic changes of pregnancy serve to aggravate the underlying pathophysiology of cardiac disorders, patients are at relatively high risk to develop congestive failure, atrial fibrillation, and supraventricular tachycardia. One in four will develop symptoms of cardiac decompensation during pregnancy. Initial therapy consists of bedrest. If this does not suffice, judicious use of digoxin and diuretics may be required. Epidural anesthesia during labor and delivery may relieve anxiety and pain, reduce cardiac afterload, and improve cardiac function.

Mitral Insufficiency

Congestive changes tend to occur at later ages than with mitral stenosis. Therefore, most women of child-bearing age with this disorder are asymptomatic and tolerate pregnancy without difficulty. If congestive changes are present, acute deterioration and atrial fibrillation may occur and should be treated as outlined for patients with mitral stenosis. Regional anesthesia is recommended.

Aortic Stenosis

High maternal and fetal mortality rates have been reported in the past. Pregnant women with this lesion rarely develop congestive failure, but angina often occurs more frequently. Patients have difficulty maintaining cardiac output in the face of acute increases in afterload or decreases in preload. Therefore, hypertension, fluid overload, and hypotension due to blood loss or regional anesthesia must be avoided.

Aortic Insufficiency

Most patients with this lesion tolerate pregnancy without difficulty. However, congestive failure occasionally occurs requiring rest, digoxin, and diuretics. Regional anesthesia is recommended for labor and delivery.

Pulmonary and Tricuspid Lesions

These lesions are rare and usually well tolerated during pregnancy. However, patients with symptomatic pulmonary stenosis are at substantially increased risk and should undergo corrective surgery prior to attempting pregnancy.

Atrial Septal Defect, Ventricular Septal Defect, Patent Ductus Arteriosus

Patients usually tolerate pregnancy without substantial deterioration unless right to left shunting and pulmonary hypertension are present. Bacterial endocarditis prophylaxis is required for VSD and PDA but not for ASD.

Pulmonary Hypertension, Eisenmenger's Syndrome

Pregnancy is contraindicated because maternal mortality is 30-50%.

Mitral Valve Prolapse

Patients with mitral valve prolapse alone usually do well during pregnancy. The prevalence of arrhythmias is increased and 20% require propranolol to control this problem. The need for prophylactic antibiotics for an uncomplicated labor and delivery is controversial.

Idiopathic Hypertrophic Subaortic Stenosis

The hemodynamic changes associated with pregnancy often result in a decrease in outflow obstruction and improvement in symptoms. However, situations predisposing to catecholamine release (pain and anxiety, hypotension due to blood loss or regional anesthesia) may aggravate symptoms during labor and should be avoided.

Coarctation of the Aorta

Patients with this disorder may be separated into complicated or uncomplicated categories on the basis of the presence or absence of associated cardiac valvular lesions. Patients with uncomplicated coarctation usually do well during pregnancy. However, gravidas with complicated coarctation are at higher risk due to potential rupture of associated intracranial aneurysms and/or aortic dissection. Therapy for the latter group consists of control of hypertension, rest, and beta-blockers as prophylaxis against dissection.

Marfan's Syndrome

Patients with an aortic arch >4.0 cm in diameter or with cardiac decompensation are at high risk for sustaining a ruptured aortic aneurysm and/or further cardiac deterioration. Pregnancy is contraindicated in such women. Gravida with an aortic arch diameter <4.0 cm and no cardiac decompensation are at relatively low risk. They should rest frequently, and beta-blockers may be considered to reduce pulse pressure.

Thromboembolic Disease

The physiologic changes of pregnancy increase the chances that a pregnant woman may experience Virchow's classic triad of factors predisposing to thrombosis: alteration in the composition of the blood, venous stasis, and vessel wall injury. During the antepartum period, the prevalence of deep vein thrombophlebitis remains similar to that found in non-pregnant women but increases by four- to sixfold during labor, delivery, and postpartum. Additionally, pulmonary embolism occurs at a rate of 0.5-12 per 1,000 deliveries. Respiratory and cardiovascular compromise as a result of this medical complication are common causes of maternal mortality, especially in the postpartum cesarean patient.

The diagnosis of thrombophlebitis is often obscured due to musculoskeletal pain and edema common in normal pregnancy. Doppler flow studies, impedance plethysmography, and limited venography may be diagnostic. Once the diagnosis is established, anticoagulant therapy has been demonstrated to decrease the probability of pulmonary embolus and result in decreased mortality. Because of the potential teratogenic and late fetal complications associated with warfarin therapy, heparin is the preferred anticoagulant during the antepartum period. It may be administered as a 70 U/kg intravenous bolus followed by an infusion of 300-400 U/kg/24 hr, or a 5,000 U bolus followed by a maintenance dose of approximately 1,000 U/hr. The maintenance infusion should be titrated to achieve a partial thromboplastin time (PTT) of 50-75 seconds or a heparin level of 0.2-0.4 U/ml. Intravenous therapy should be continued for 7-10 days. In the postpartum period, warfarin therapy may be initiated and continued for three months. In the antepartum period, a moderate dose of subcutaneous heparin (approximately 10,000 U b.i.d. or 7,000 U t.i.d. adjusted to maintain a therapeutic PTT or heparin level) may be administered for three months followed by a subcutaneous dose of 5,000 U b.i.d. for the remainder of the pregnancy.

Unfortunately, laboratory studies to diagnose a pulmonary embolism (Table 2.6) are usually insensitive and nonspecific. If clinical suspicion of a pulmonary embolus is high and certain diagnostic tests are delayed or inconclusive, intravenous heparin therapy should be initiated in the dosage outlined above. Once the diagnosis is confirmed, long term therapy should be utilized according to the above guidelines for a minimum of 3-6 months. If emboli recur after adequate anticoagulation, vena cava ligation should be considered.

Women who have experienced a thromboembolic event before pregnancy appear to have a 12% recurrence risk. This observation has led us to administer a minidose of subcutaneous heparin (5,000 U q 12 h) to such gravidas from the 34th week of gestation until the patients are fully ambulatory postpartum. Some investigators have recommended that this practice be extended to other high risk groups including women with advanced maternal age, high parity, obesity, immobility, diabetes, hypertension, cardiac disease, or severe varicose veins.

Drug Abuse

Many questions that patients ask about drugs relate to illicit or "street" drug use in early pregnancy. Although the risk of fetal malformation with inadvertant use in early gestation is unknown, no benefit from continued use is possible, and premature delivery is more likely. Furthermore, the effect of these drugs (which readily cross

Table 2.6
Tests Used to Diagnose a Pulmonary Embolus

Test	Findings Suggestive of Pulmonary Embolus	Aids to Differential Diagnosis	Therapeutic Implication
Arterial blood gases	Low pO_2 and low or normal pCO_2 are nearly constant findings	Normal pO_2 nearly excludes	Guide to oxygen therapy and prognosis
Chest x-ray	Enlargement of main pulmonary artery and right ventricle, lung infiltrate, pleural effusion, elevated diaphragm, or asymmetry of vasculature	To rule out pneumonia and congestive heart failure (may be secondary)	Presence of acute right ventricular enlargement indicates life-threatening embolism
ECG	Right axis shift and right ventricular strain	To rule out acute myocardial infarction or ischemia	Detection and treatment of arrhythmia
Ventilation/perfusion scan (V/Q)	Areas of oligemia (areas of the lung with a decreased concentration of radioactivity on perfusion studies with unmatched areas on ventilation)	Equivocal scan can be caused by pneumonia, atelectasis, or other pulmonary lesions	Extent of V/Q mismatch serves as a guide to severity
Pulm. angiogram	Filling defects distally	Normal angiogram excludes large emboli, cutoffs of pulmonary arteries, areas of decreased perfusion	Most accurate guide to assess

the placenta) on fetal neurobehavioral development cannot be assessed with certainty.

Cocaine use has gained recent nationwide attention and is the most commonly abused substance of most pregnant drug addicts. Preliminary observations have suggested that there is a significantly higher rate of spontaneous abortion, growth retardation, stillbirth, and malformation. Infants exposed in utero to cocaine are also more likely to show depressed interactive behavior with poor organizational response to environmental stimuli. A broader assessment requiring larger numbers of pregnancies and longer follow-up is necessary for more definitive impressions.

Most persons will discontinue these drug habits once pregnancy is diagnosed. Abortion is not recommended for drug exposure alone. Tests of amniotic fluid are not available which will assess fetal involvement. Listed below are general recommendations for assessing the mother and fetus and for management of drug dependency.

Baseline Laboratory Studies

1. Complete blood count with indices
2. Blood smear
3. Urine culture (minimum of two during pregnancy)
4. Tuberculin skin test
5. Folic acid level
6. Total protein - A/G ratio
7. Liver function profile
8. Rubella titer
9. Serologic test for syphilis (RPR, VDRL, etc.)
10. Gonorrhea culture (cervical) of initial visit and repeat at 36 weeks
11. HBsAg (Hepatitis B surface antigen)
12. Pap smear
13. Blood type, Rh, and irregular antibody screen
14. Ultrasound scan
15. Herpes culture (if positive history)
16. Sickle cell prep (if anemia and black)
17. Serum HIV antibody titer (after permission)

Nutrition

1. Diet consultation
2. Ingestion of fresh fruit, fresh vegetables, lean meats, dairy products
3. Prevent deficiency states
4. Prevent maternal urine ketosis
5. Frequent complete blood counts
6. Diet recall with each visit
7. Assess dental hygiene
8. Encourage smoking cessation

Infection

1. Examine for and treat any sexually transmitted disease
2. Screen for hepatitis B
3. Watch for and treat any other illness
4. Examine urine for infection
5. Search for preexisting bacterial endocarditis

Psychosocial

1. Establish contact with social services for care before and after delivery and for infant placement (if necessary)
2. Watch for suicidal depression (hospitalize without delay)

Drug Management

1. Watch for multiple drug use (including alcohol). May need to perform urine drug screens intermittently
2. Supportive withdrawal: minor tranquilizers and sedatives, amphetamines, tobacco
3. Maintenance therapy for narcotic abuse: gradual detoxification with oral methadone, usually beginning with approximately 40 mg daily; decrease methadone dose (2 mg/week) with caution and attempt to achieve 20 mg/day or less by delivery to minimize any neonatal withdrawal

Fetal Assessment

1. No tests of amniotic fluid to assess fetal effects from drugs or a karyotype analysis are recommended
2. Serial ultrasound examinations to search for IUGR
3. Perform fetal well-being tests in third trimester
4. Notify pediatrician before labor and delivery
5. Use of nalaxone (Narcan) is contraindicated in newborns of drug addicted mothers, since it may initiate an immediate withdrawal syndrome. Support any respiratory depression with mechanical ventilation
6. Effects from specific abused drugs on the mother and fetus are shown in Table 2.7.

Table 2.7
Effects from Specific Abused Drugs

Drug Groups	Maternal Signs and Symptoms of Overdose	Maternal Withdrawal Symptoms	Fetal/Neonatal Effects
Alcohol	Unusual behavior; mostly depressant with stupor, loss of memory, hypotension	Agitation, tremors	Microcephaly, mental retardation, facial dysmorphia, failure to thrive
Marijuana	Pupils normal but conjunctiva injected	None	None known; meconium during labor (?)
CNS Sedatives (barbiturates, chlordiazepoxide, diazepam, flurazepam, methaqualone)	Pupils fixed, BP decreased, respiration depressed, reflexes hypoactive, drowsiness, coma, lateral nystagmus, slurred speech, delirium, convulsions	Tremulousness, insomnia, chronic blink reflex, agitation, toxic psychosis	Decreased heart variability; sedation or respiratory depression (mild if present)
CNS Stimulants (cocaine antiobesity drugs, amphetamines)	Pupils dilated and reactive, respirations shallow, BP increased, reflexes hyperactive	Muscle aches, abdominal pain, hunger, prolonged sleep, suicidal	Hyperactivity with increased kicks; spont. abortion (?) premature labor (?)
Hallucinogens (LSD, phencyclidine)	Pupils dilated, BP elevated, heart rate increased, reflexes hyperactive, face flushed, euphoria, anxiety, inappropriate affect, illusions, hallucinations	No withdrawal symptoms	No known fetal effects; behavior problems, facial abnormalities (?)

Table 2.7 (Continued)

Drug Groups	Maternal Signs and Symptoms of Overdose	Maternal Withdrawal Symptoms	Fetal/Neonatal Effects
Narcotics (codeine, heroin, meperidine, morphine, opium)	Pupils constricted, respiration and BP decreased, reflexes hypo-active, sensorium obtunded	Flu-like syndrome, agitation, dilated pupils abdominal pain	Intrauterine withdrawal with increased fetal activity, newborn withdrawal, increased rates of IUGR and IUFD
Solvents (glue, gas-oline, clean-ing solutions)	Euphoria, toxicity to liver and kidneys	Agitation	"Fetal Solvent Syndrome" (?) (similar to alcohol syndrome)

Seizure Disorders

Seizure disorders are found in approximately 1 in 100 pregnant women. Several years were required to recognize the teratogenic potential of most anticonvulsant medications because of the compounding effects of metabolic changes, seizure-related hypoxia, and genetic factors. Current therapy requires prescribing a minimal number of medications with the least teratogenic potential using the lowest dose compatible with maternal seizure control.

Before Conception

An understanding of the type of seizure disorder and any medications taken is necessary. Table 2.8 lists drug therapy for specific seizure disorders. Most patients requiring long-term drug therapy have grand mal or tonic-clonic seizures. The risk to an unborn child of developing epilepsy is 2-3% or 5 times greater than the general population. A patient should not be discouraged from becoming pregnant unless the seizures are difficult to control, causing her to be incapable of responsible parenting. The risk of a seizure disorder worsening during the pregnancy is 50%, being unaltered is 5%, and improving is 45%. This risk is greater if seizures have occurred recently.

Anticonvulsant drugs may be withdrawn several months before conception if the patient has been seizure-free for several years, has a recent normal EEG, and can be followed closely. The least number of anticonvulsant medications is recommended, and phenobarbital is the single most preferred drug. Discontinuing or substituting for trimethadione and valproic acid should be done before or shortly after

Table 2.8
Drug Therapy for Specific Seizure Disorders during Pregnancy

Seizure Disorder	Primary Drug	Secondary Drug
Grand mal (tonic-clonic)	Phenobarbital	Phenytoin Carbamazepine Primidone
Psychomotor	Primidone	Phenytoin Phenobarbital Carbamazepine
Petit mal (absence)	Ethosuximide	Clonazepam
Status epilepticus	Diazepam followed by phenytoin	Phenytoin Phenobarbital Paraldehyde Thiopental

conception, since the teratogenic potential is of greater concern than seizure control.

Antepartum Management

When possible, the patient should be switched to phenobarbital in the preconception period. If the patient is already pregnant, medications used to control grand mal seizures before pregnancy should be continued rather than withdrawn. Prior neurologic evaluations and any test results should be obtained.

Adverse effects on the mother and fetus for each anticonvulsant are uncommon but are listed in Table 2.9. The risk of fetal anomalies in pregnant women on anticonvulsant therapy is 2-3 times greater than the general population, and the risk of mental retardation is perhaps slightly greater using these drugs. However, a greater risk is presented to the fetus by prolonged hypoxia from a grand mal seizure or from unconsciousness.

Serum drug levels ("free" or unbound fraction) should be obtained monthly during the antepartum period. The dosage frequently needs to be increased during pregnancy to maintain therapeutic levels of at least one of the drugs. (Table 2.10). It is quite uncommon for more than two anticonvulsants (phenytoin and phenobarbitol) to be taken during pregnancy.

Petit mal seizures are rare in adults. Whether patients with petit mal or psychomotor seizure disorders should continue their medications during pregnancy is unclear. Consultation with a neurologist is recommended.

Table 2.9
Adverse Maternal and Fetal Effects from Anticonvulsant Use

Maternal	Fetal/Neonatal
Phenytoin (Dilantin) Cardiovascular collapse after rapid IV injection, ataxia, nystagmus, GI upset, increased incidence of seizures, behavioral changes	Probable teratogenicity, neonatal coagulopathy, hypocalcemia and tetany
Phenobarbital Drowsiness (transient), ataxia, respiratory depression, sleep abnormalities, hypotension, withdrawal	Possible low-level teratogenicity, neonatal depression, coagulopathy and hemorrhage
Primidone (Mysoline) Ataxia, vertigo, headache, nausea morbilliform rash, nystagmus	Possible teratogenicity, neonatal coagulopathy and depression
Carbamazepine (Tegretol) Diplopia, drowsiness, leukopenia, transient blurred vision, rash, disturbance of equilibrium	None known
Ethosuximide (Zarontin) Hematopoietic complications Changes in the liver, GI upset, nausea, vomiting, diarrhea, behavioral changes	Possible low-level teratogenicity
Valproic acid GI upset, sedation, ataxia, loss of coordination, hepatotoxicity, and thrombocytopenia	Open neural tube defects
Trimethadione (Tridione) Sedation, blurred vision in bright light, nonspecific GI and neurologic effects, skin rashes, lupus syndrome	Definite teratogenicity
Diazepam (Valium) Depressed respiration, bradycardia, hypotension, cardiovascular collapse, paradoxical hyperexcitability, withdrawal	Possible low level teratogenicity, decreased fetal heart rate variability, neonatal depression, withdrawal, impaired thermoregulation

Table 2.10
Daily Dosages of Specific Anticonvulsant to Maintain Therapeutic
Serum Levels

Drug	Adult Daily Dosage (mg)	Therapeutic Level (mcg/ml)
Phenytoin (Dilantin)	300-500	10-20
Phenobarbital	90-120	15-40
Carbamazepine (Tegretol)	800-1,200	4-16
Primidone (Mysoline)	750-1,500	5-15

Folic acid (1 mg) should be given to any patient taking phenytoin, phenobarbital, or primidone (all folic acid antagonists) to perhaps decrease the incidence of birth defects. This dose is present in most standard prenatal vitamins. The measurement of serum folate levels is unnecessary. Pregnant epileptics receiving phenytoin, phenobarbital, or primidone should be given oral vitamin K (5-10 mg/d) during the last month of pregnancy. This should bypass any decrease in synthesis of vitamin K-dependent clotting factors caused by these drugs.

Status epilepticus should be treated vigorously regardless of the pregnancy. Diazepam (Valium) 10 mg should be administerd intravenously over 1-3 min after the patient's airway is opened and free exchange of air takes place. Phenytoin (Dilantin) 200-500 mg is then given intravenously depending on anticonvulsant blood levels.

Intrapartum/Postpartum Management

The pediatric staff should be notified of any impending delivery. Evidence of fetal malformations or neonatal depression and withdrawal should be sought in infants born to mothers taking phenytoin, phenobarbital, or primidone. Coagulation studies of the cord blood should be performed and the infant should be given 1 mg of vitamin K IM shortly after birth.

Intravenous anticonvulsant therapy using Dilantin (500 mg IV over 1/2 hr every 12 hrs) or magnesium sulfate (1-2 gm/hr) should be continued during labor unless progress is rapid. Dilantin should not be mixed in a dextrose-containing solution, because intravenous crystalization may occur.

Breast feeding is permissible if no infant signs of depression are evident. Anticonvulsant drug doses should be decreased after delivery according to serum drug levels.

Thyroid Disease

Hyperthyroidism

Next to diabetes, untreated or previously treated hyperthyroidism is the most common endocrine disorder encountered during pregnacy. As signs and symptoms of thyroid hyperfunction are similar to certain patient complaints during pregnancy, and thyroid tests are altered by pregnancy-induced changes in serum proteins, the diagnosis of hyperthyroidism is often difficult. However, therapy is necessary to avoid maternal and fetal complications. If untreated, stillbirth rates are increased to 8-15%, and premature delivery may occur in up to one-fourth of affected patients.

Drug treatment of hyperthyroidism during pregnancy is intended to decrease the amount of circulating thyroid hormones and to relieve bothersome symptoms. A subtotal thyroidectomy is rarely indicated and only if there is failed medical management, inadequate patient compliance, or need for excessive medication. Therapeutic radioactive iodine is contraindicated because of its damaging effects on the fetal thyroid gland; abortion is not recommended if therapy was discontinued two months or more before conception.

The two principle antithyroid drugs, propylthiouracil and methimazole, act to prevent iodination of tyrosine by inhibiting the oxidation of iodide to iodine. Impairment of the peripheral conversion of thyroxine (T_4) to triiodothyronine (T_3) is also seen within the first few days of therapy.

Response to therapy may take up to 6 weeks, since present thyroid hormone stores need to be depleted. Adjustment of dosage after that time is dependent on circulating levels of free T_4 or free thyroxine index (FTI) as well as patient symptoms. Free T_4 or FTI levels should be maintained within an upper normal or slightly elevated range during pregnancy. If the patient is already on this medication at the time of conception, there is thought to be no added risk of teratogenesis. The medication may be tapered or discontinued depending on patient symptoms.

Propylthiouracil in 50-mg tablets is preferred over methimazole, since fewer adverse effects may be found in the infant. A beginning dose of 100-150 mg t.i.d. or b.i.d. should be cut in half after 3-4 weeks if testing indicates improved thyroid function. A usual daily maintenance dose is 100 mg (50 mg b.i.d.) and should not exceed 300 mg, since this medication crosses the placenta and may cause fetal hypothyroidism. The pediatrician should be notified of this situation before delivery, since hypothyroidism in the newborn may last for a few days until the drug is eliminated.

Symptoms relating to enhanced sympathomimetic activity such as tremors, tachycardia, and palpitations are seen in patients with hyperthyroidism. A beta-blocker such as propranolol may be used when symptoms are severe. This drug is also used in patients with hypertension, mitral valve prolapse, and severe migraine headaches. Because of its beta-blocking action, there may be a loss of beat-to-beat variability, bradycardia, hypoglycemia, and transient respiratory depression in the newborn and it should be discontinued shortly before delivery to minimize peripartum drug effects.

Thyroid storm occurs rarely during pregnancy most commonly in patients with no history of thyroid disease. It is characterized by a high fever (103°F or more), tachycardia, nausea and vomiting, or central nervous system involvement and is usually precipitated by infection, ketoacidosis, or surgery. Therapy for the pregnant patient with thyroid storm includes the following: copious intravenous fluids, propranolol (40 mg p.o. q 6 h or 1-2 mg IV slowly until pulse rate less than 100 beats/min), propylthiouracil (300 mg p.o. q 6 h), hydrocortisone (100 mg IV q 8 h) sodium iodide (1 gm IV), hypothermia induction.

Thyroid function should be monitored carefully in the first few postpartum months, since severe and unpredictable alterations in thyroid function may occur. The IgG immunoglobulin, LATS (long-acting thyroid stimulator), in mothers with Graves' disease can cross the placenta easily and remain within the newborn's circulation.

Hypothyroidism

Hypothyroidism is found most commonly after a subtotal thyroidectomy. Affected patients have symptoms similar to usual complaints during pregnancy which include fatigueability and cold intolerance. Most patients are on thyroid replacement therapy at conception. This medication should be continued during pregnancy, since documented hypothyroidism may be associated with an increased risk of an unfavorable perinatal outcome and thyroid hormone reserves will become further depleted.

The amount of thyroid supplementation required is titrated upward until serum TSH has returned to normal (less than 10 mIU/ml). Levothyroxine (Synthroid) is the preferred drug during pregnancy. The 0.05-0.1 mg tablets taken daily contain 100 mg of thyroxine which is then peripherally converted to thyronine. This drug is the most physiologic replacement available and does not cross the placenta because of its physicochemical properties.

The only major maternal complication associated with thyroid supplementation is overdosage with resulting signs of hyperthyroidism. Along with monitoring clinical signs, periodic TSH determinations should be obtained. Serum free thyroid hormone levels may be falsely elevated. Thyroid function should be monitored carefully in the first few postpartum months, since severe and unpredictable alterations in thyroid function may occur.

Collagen Vascular Disease

Rheumatoid arthritis and systemic lupus erythematosus are the most common collagen vascular disorders and perhaps the most amenable to treatment. Approximately three-fourths of women with rheumatoid arthritis experience symptomatic improvement during pregnancy, and the condition does not apparently cause a deleterious effect on the pregnancy.

Salicylates form the mainstay of drug therapy for rheumatoid arthritis. They exert their antiinflammatory effect by blocking prostaglandin synthesis. Enteric-coated aspirin is preferred. Salicylates cross the placenta easily, but the overwhelming body of information has not demonstrated teratogenic effects. The length of gestation is thought to be increased with a higher incidence of post-dates pregnancies, and duration of labor is more prolonged in women being treated with these prostaglandin inhibiting drugs. Maternal salicylate ingestion is also associated with a greater chance of neonatal platelet dysfunction. Intracranial hemorrhage among infants may also be more common during the delivery process.

Other nonsteroidal prostaglandin synthetase inhibiting (PGSI) drugs have been utilized in patients with rheumatoid arthritis. These medicines have also been used for the prevention of premature labor in several investigational trials. Ductus arteriosus closure in the fetus with subsequent pulmonary hypertension is a potential concern, and use of these agents is not encouraged during the pregnancy.

The course of lupus during pregnancy is more variable. Flare-ups are usually reduced dramatically, but exacerbation of nephritis is particularly dangerous and difficult to differentiate from preeclampsia. Patients with lupus experience a greater hazard of spontaneous abortion and stillbirth, and some studies have reported an increased risk of fetal growth retardation and prematurity.

Corticosteroid therapy is the principal drug for treatment of systemic lupus. The lowest dose to relieve symptoms and prevent recurrence is desired. A 20-40 mg daily dose of prednisone may be used for flares with non-major organ involvement. Evidence of nephritis, cerebritis, or vasculitis requires an increase in the dose to 40-80 mg. The only controlled study of the use of corticosteroids revealed that those patients had fewer exacerbations and less perinatal mortality than those who did not receive corticosteroids.

The lack of knowledge about agents such as immunosuppressive medications, penicillamine, and gold during pregnancy would warrant that they be avoided except in life threatening situations.

Asthma

Asthma occurs in approximately 1% of all pregnant patients. The prognosis is unpredictable, but most women generally do well with cautious surveillance and proper medical therapy. Approximately 10% of gravidas with asthma require hospitalization for acute attacks. An increased frequency of prematurity, low birth weight, stillbirth, and neonatal neurologic abnormalities has been reported in asthmatics compared with those without asthma.

Many drugs are available for the control of asthma, and therapy differs little from non-pregnancy. The intermittent inhalation of beta-agonists (albuterol or metaproterenol), two deep inhalations every 4-6 hours, may be all that is necessary. Oral methylxanthine therapy should be initiated if the inhalation therapy is inadequate. Aminophylline (200-300 mg four times daily) or Theodur (200 mg every 12 hours) may be used. Serum drug levels should be maintained within a therapeutic range (10-20 mg/ml). Methylxanthines inhibit the force of uterine contractions, and prolonged gestation or long labor may occur. Acceleration of fetal lung development may also occur because of their phosphodiesterase-inhibiting property.

Corticosteroid therapy using a single daily oral dose of Prednisone (60-100 mg) is recommended for women with refractory symptoms. If improvement occurs within six hours, the dose is usually tapered over the next few weeks. A 100 mg intravenous dose of hydrocortisone should be given every 12 hours during labor and immediately postpartum if prolonged corticosteroid therapy has been necessary.

Inflammatory Bowel Disease

Ulcerative colitis and regional enteritis usually begin in adolescence or early adulthood when reproductive capabilities begin. With modern management techniques neither bowel disorder appears to be associated with an increased maternal-fetal or neonatal complication rate. Recent reports also suggest that there is no increase in the frequency of exacerbation during pregnancy.

Therapy for inflammatory bowel disease usually involves the modification of the diet to avoid vegetables, certain fruits, and lactulose. Calcium intake should be supplemented with over-the-counter products as Os-Cal, 1-2 tablets three times daily. Codeine and Immodium are probably not associated with any increased fetal risk but should be used judiciously during pregnancy. Other constipating agents such as Metamucil, Pepto-bismol, and Amphojel may be preferable. Corticosteroids are usually prescribed when the above measures fail. No increase in fetal or neonatal complications has been attributed to corticosteroid therapy.

Sulfasalazine is also used frequently with corticosteroid therapy. Prolonged treatment for the prevention of recurrence is thought to be of little benefit, but a 2-6 gm oral dose daily is helpful for acute attacks. No teratogenic effect has been attributed to this medication. Being a sulfur preparation, sulfasalazine is theorized to be associated with displacement of bilirubin from albumin molecules and neonatal jaundice. This complication is thought to be very uncommon, however. Very little information has been published about azathioprine for treatment of inflammatory bowel disease during pregnancy.

Suggested Readings

Gestational Diabetes

Lavin JP, Barden TP, Miodovnik M: Clinical experience with a screening program for gestational diabetes. Am. J. Obstet. Gynecol. 141:491, 1981.

Shah BD, Cohen AW, May C, et al: Comparison of glycohemoglobin determination and the one-hour oral glucose screen in the identification of gestational diabetes. Am. J. Obstet. Gynecol. 144:774, 1982.

Cousins L, Dattel B, Hollingsworth D, et al: Screening for carbohydrate intolerance in pregnancy: A comparison of two tests and reassessment of a common approach. Am. J. Obstet. Gynecol. 153:381, 1985.

Grant PT, Oats JN, Beischer N: The long-term follow-up of women with gestational diabetes. Aust. N.Z. J. Obstet, Gynaecol. 26:17, 1986.

Gabbe SG: Definition, detection, and management of gestational diabetes. Obstet. Gynecol. 67:121, 1986.

Coustan DR, Widness JA, Carpenter MW, et al: Should the fifty-gram, one-hour plasma glucose screening test for gestational diabetes be administered in the fasting or fed state? Am. J. Obstet. Gynecol. 154:1031, 1986.

Blumenthal SA, Abdul-Karim RW: Diagnosis, classification, and metabolic management of diabetes in pregnancy: Therapeutic impact of self-monitoring of blood glucose and of newer methods of insulin delivery. Obstet. & Gynecol. Surv. 42:593, 1987.

Bochner CJ, Medearis AL, Williams J, et al: Early third-trimester ultrasound screening in gestational diabetes to determine the risk of macrosomia and labor dystocia at term. Am. J. Obstet. Gynecol. 157:703, 1987.

Weiner CP, Faustich MW, Burns J, et al: Diagnosis of gestational diabetes by capillary blood samples and a portable reflectance meter: Derivation of threshold values and prospective validation. Am. J. Obstet. Gynecol. 156:1085, 1987.

Langer O, Anyaegbunam A, Brustman L, et al: Gestational diabetes: Insulin requirements in pregnancy. Am. J. Obstet. Gynecol. 157:669, 1987.

Position statement on gestational diabetes mellitus. Am. J. Obstet. Gynecol. 156:488, 1987.

Main EK, Main DM, Gabbe SG: Chronic oral terbutaline tocolytic therapy is associated with maternal glucose intolerance. Am. J. Obstet. Gynecol. 157:644, 1987.

Insulin-Dependent Diabetes

Golde SH, Good-Anderson B, Montoro M, et al: Insulin requirements during labor: A reappraisal. Am. J. Obstet. Gynecol. 144:556, 1982.

Hollingsworth DR: Alterations of maternal metabolism in normal and diabetic pregnancies: Differences in insulin-dependent, non-insulin-dependent, and gestational diabetes. Am. J. Obstet. Gynecol. 146:417, 1983.

Ferroni KM, Gross TL, Sokol RJ, et al: What affects fetal pulmonary maturation during diabetic pregnancy? Am. J. Obstet. Gynecol. 150:270, 1984.

Golde SH, Montoro M, Good-Anderson B, et al: The role of nonstress tests, fetal biophysical profile, and contraction stress tests in the outpatient management of insulin-requiring diabetic pregnancies. Am. J. Obstet. Gynecol. 148:269, 1984.

Warram JH, Krolewski AS, Gottlieb MS, et al: Differences in risk of insulin-dependent diabetes in offspring of diabetic mothers and diabetic fathers. N. Engl. J. Med. 311:149, 1984.

Miodovnik M, Lavin JP, Knowles HC, et al: Spontaneous abortion among insulin-dependent diabetic women. Am. J. Obstet. Gynecol. 150:372, 1984.

Freinkel N, Dooley SL, Metzger BE: Care of the pregnant woman with insulin-dependent diabetes mellitus. N. Engl. J. Med. 313:96, 1985.

Kitzmiller JL, Younger MD, Hare JW, et al: Continuous subcutaneous insulin therapy during early pregnancy. Obstet Gynecol. 66:606, 1985.

Sutherland HW, Pritchard CW: Increased incidence of spontaneous abortion in pregnancies complicated by maternal diabetes mellitus. Am. J. Obstet. Gynecol. 155:135, 1986.

Centers for Disease Control Morbidity and Mortality Weekly Report. 35, April 4, 1986.

Reece EA, Hobbins JC: Diabetic embryopathy: Pathogenesis, prenatal diagnosis and prevention. Obstet. & Gynecol. Surv. 41:325, 1986.

Management of diabetes mellitus in pregnancy. ACOG Tech. Bull. 92, May, 1986.

Landon MB, Gabbe SG, Piana R, et al: Neonatal morbidity in pregnancy complicated by diabetes mellitus: Predictive value of maternal glycemic profiles. Am. J. Obstet. Gynecol. 156:1089, 1987.

Cousins L: Pregnancy complications among diabetic women: Review 1965-1985. Obstet. & Gynecol. Surv. 42:140, 1987.

Mimouni F, Miodovnik M, Whitsett JA, et al: Respiratory distress syndrome in infants of diabetic mothers in the 1980s: No direct adverse effect of maternal diabetes with modern management. Obstet. Gynecol. 69:191, 1987.

Blumenthal SA, Abdul-Karim RW: Diagnosis, classification, and metabolic management of diabetes in pregnancy: Therapeutic impact of self-monitoring of blood glucose and of newer methods of insulin delivery. Obstet. & Gynecol. Surv. 42:592, 1987.

Obesity

Peckham CH, Christianson RE: The relationship between prepregnancy weight and certain obstetric factors. Am. J. Obstet. Gynecol. 111:1, 1971.

Freedman MA, Wilds PL, George WM: Grotesque obesity: A serious complication of labor and delivery. Southern Med. J. 65:732, 1972.

Maeder EC, Barno A, Mecklenburg F: Obesity: A maternal high-risk factor. Obstet. Gynecol. 45:669, 1975.

Edwards LE, Dickes WF, Alton IR, et al: Pregnancy in the massively obese: Course, outcome, and obesity prognosis of the infant. Am. J. Obstet. Gynecol. 131:479, 1978.

Cohen AW, Gabbe SG: When obesity complicates pregnancy. Contemp. Ob/Gyn 15:45, 1980.

Kliegman RM, Gross T: Perinatal problems of the obese mother and her infant. Obstet. Gynecol. 66:299, 1985.

Algert S, Shragg P, Hollingsworth DR: Moderate caloric restriction in obese women with gestational diabetes. Obstet. Gynecol. 65:487, 1985.

Garbaciak JA, Richter M, Miller S, et al: Maternal weight and pregnancy complications. Am. J. Obstet. Gynecol. 152:238, 1985.

Chronic Hypertension

Chesley LC: Hypertension in pregnancy: Definitions, familial factor, and remote prognosis. Kidney Int. 18:234, 1980.

Sibai BM, Abdella TN, Anderson GD, et al: Plasma volume findings in pregnant women with mild hypertension: Therapeutic considerations. Am. J. Obstet. Gynecol. 145:439, 1983.

Sibai BM, Abdella TN, Anderson GD: Pregnancy outcome in 211 patients with mild chronic hypertension. Obstet. Gynecol. 61:571, 1983.

Lindheimer MD, Katz AI: Hypertension in pregnancy. N. Engl. J. Med. 313:6515, 1985.

Sibai BM, Anderson GD: Pregnancy outcome of intensive therapy in severe hypertension in first trimester. Obstet. Gynecol. 67:517, 1986.

Weitz C, Khouzami V, Maxwell K, et al: Treatment of hypertension in pregnancy with methyldopa: A randomized double blind study. Int. J. Gynaecol. Obstet. 25:35, 1987.

Pregnancy-Induced Hypertension

Ounsted M, Cockburn J, Moar VA, et al: Maternal hypertension with superimposed preeclampsia: Effects on child development at 7 1/2 years. Br. J. Obstet. Gynaecol. 90:644, 1983.

Svensson A, Andersch B, Hansson L: A clinical follow-up study of 260 women with hypertension in pregnancy. Clin. Exp. Hypertens. 2:95, 1983.

Campbell DM, MacGillivray I, Carr-Hill R: Pre-eclampsia in second pregnancy. Br. J. Obstet. Gynaecol. 92:131, 1985.

Management of preeclampsia. ACOG Tech. Bull. 91, February, 1986.

Rote NS, Harrison M, Lau RJ, et al: Thrombocytopenia in pregnancy-induced hypertension: IgG and IgM on maternal and umbilical cord platelets. Obstet. Gynecol. Surv. 42:291, 1987.

Severe Preeclampsia or Eclampsia

Pritchard JA, Cunningham FG, Mason RA: Coagulation changes in eclampsia: Their frequency and pathogenesis. Am. J. Obstet. Gynecol. 124:855, 1976.

Weinstein L: Syndrome of hemolysis, elevated liver enzymes, and low platelet count: A severe consequence of hypertension in pregnancy. Am. J. Obstet. Gynecol. 142:159, 1982.

Sibai BM, Anderson GD, Abdella TN, et al: Eclampsia III. Neonatal outcome, growth, and development. Am. J. Obstet. Gynecol. 146:307, 1983.

Henderson DW, VilosGA, Milne KJ, et al: The role of Swan-Ganz catheterization in severe pregnancy-induced hypertension. Am. J. Obstet. Gynecol. 148:570, 1984.

Pritchard JA, Cunningham FG, Pritchard SA: The Parkland Memorial Hospital protocol for treatment of eclampsia: Evaluation of 245 cases. Am. J. Obstet. Gynecol. 148:951, 1984.

Sibai BM, Spinnato JA, Watson DL, et al: Pregnancy outcome in 303 cases with severe preeclampsia. Obstet. Gynecol. 64:319, 1984.

Cotton DB, Gonik B, Dorman K, et al: Cardiovascular alterations in severe pregnancy-induced hypertension: Relationship of central venous pressure to pulmonary capillary wedge pressure. Am. J. Obstet. Gynecol. 151:762, 1985.

Sibai BM, Spinnato JA, Watson DL, et al: Eclampsia IV. Neurological findings and future outcome. Am. J. Obstet. Gynecol. 152:184, 1985.

Sibai BM, Taslimi MM, El-Nazer A, et al: Maternal-perinatal outcome associated with the syndrome of hemolysis, elevated liver enzymes, and low platelets in severe preeclampsia-eclampsia. Am. J. Obstet. Gynecol. 155:501, 1986.

Cardiac Disorders

Rayburn WF, Fontana ME: Mitral valve prolapse and pregnancy. Am. J. Obstet. Gynecol. 141:9, 1981.

Sugrue D, Blake S, MacDonald D: Pregnancy complicated by maternal heart disease at the National Maternity Hospital, Dublin, Ireland, 1969 to 1978. Am. J. Obstet. Gynecol. 139:1, 1981.

Payne DG, Fishburne JI, Rufty AJ, et al: Bacterial endocarditis in pregnancy. Obstet. Gynecol. 60:247, 1982.

Tamari I, Eldar M, Rabinowitz B, et al: Medical treatment of cardiovascular disorders during pregnancy. Am. Heart J. 104:1357, 1982.

Veille JC: Peripartum cardiomyopathies: A review. Am. J. Obstet. Gynecol. 148:805, 1984.

Elkayam U, Gleicher N: Cardiac problems in pregnancy. J. Am. Med. Asso. 251:2838, 1984.

Hankins GDV, Wendel GD, Leveno KJ, et al: Myocardial infarction during pregnancy: A review. Obstet. Gynecol. 65:139, 1985.

Thromboembolic Disease

Bissell SM: Pulmonary thromboembolism associated with gynecologic surgery and pregnancy. Am. J. Obstet. Gynecol. 128:418, 1977.

Clarke-Pearson DL, Creasman WT: Diagnosis of deep venous thrombosis in obstetrics and gynecology by impedance phlebography. Obstet. Gynecol. 58:52, 1981.

Bolan, JC: Thromboembolic complications of pregnancy. Clin. Obstet. Gynecol. 26:913, 1983.

Didoklar SM, Koontz C, Schimberg PI: Phleborheography in pregnancy. Obstet. Gynecol. 61:363, 1983.

Knuppel RA, Hoffman MS, O'Brien WF: Precautions on ob anticoagulant use. Contemp. Ob/Gyn. 25:53, 1985.

Lavin JP: Pharmacologic therapy for chronic medical disorders during pregnancy. In Drug Therapy in Obstetrics and Gynecology, 2nd ed., edited by WF Rayburn, FP Zuspan. East Norwalk CT, Appleton-Century-Crofts, 1986, pp 129-146.

Delclos GL, Davila F: Thrombolytic therapy for pulmonary embolism in pregnancy: A case report. Am. J. Obstet. Gynecol. 155:375, 1986.

Hux CH, Wapner RJ, Chayen B, et al: Use of the Greenfield filter for thromboembolic disease in pregnancy. Am. J. Obstet. Gynecol. 155:734, 1986.

LeClerc J, Hirsh J: Venous thromboembolic disorders. In Medical Complications during Pregnancy, edited by GN Burrow, T Ferris, ed. 3. Philadelphia, W.B. Saunders, 1988, pp 204-223.

Drug Abuse

Rosner MA, Keith L, Chasnoff I: The Northwestern University drug dependence program: The impact of intensive prenatal care on labor and delivery outcomes. Am. J. Obstet. Gynecol. 144:23, 1982.

Blinick G, Wallach RC, Jerez E, et al: Drug addiction in pregnancy and the neonate. Am. J. Obstet. Gynecol. 125:135, 1976.

Hatch EE, Bracken MB: Effect of marijuana use in pregnancy on fetal growth. Am. J. Epidemiol. 124:986, 1986.

Drug abuse and pregnancy. ACOG Tech. Bull. 96, September, 1986.

MacGregor SN, Keith LG, Chasnoff IJ, et al: Cocaine use during pregnancy: Adverse perinatal outcome. Am. J. Obstet. Gynecol. 157:686, 1987.

Woods JR, Plessinger MA, Clark KE: Effect of cocaine on uterine blood flow and fetal oxygenation. J. Am. Med. Asso. 257:957, 1987.

Seizure Disorders

Rane A, Bertilsson L, Palmer L: Disposition of placentally transferred carbamazepine (Tegretol) in the newborn. Europ. J. Clin. Pharmacol. 8:283, 1975.

Aminoff MJ: Neurological disorders and pregnancy. Am. J. Obstet. Gynecol. 132:325, 1978.

Dalessio DJ: Seizure disorders and pregnancy. N. Engl. J. Med. 312:559, 1985.

Stempel L, Rayburn W: Anticonvulsant therapy during pregnancy In Drug Therapy in Obstetrics and Gynecology, ed. 2. East Norwalk CT, Appleton-Century-Crofts, 1986, pp 53-72.

Donaldson J: Neurologic complications In Medical Complications during Pregnancy, edited by GN Burrow, T Ferris, ed. 3. Philadelphia, W.B. Saunders, 1988, pp 485-498.

Thyroid Disease

Mujtaba Q, Burrow GN: Treatment of hyperthyroidism in pregnancy with propylthiouracil and methimazole. Obstet. Gynecol. 46:282, 1975.

Burrow GN: Hyperthyroidism during pregnancy. N. Engl. J. Med. 298:150, 1978.

Kampmann JP, Hansen JM, Johansen K, et al: Propylthiouracil in human milk: Revision of a dogma. Lancet 1:736, 1980.

Sugrue D, Drury MI: Hyperthyroidism complicating pregnancy: Results of treatment by antithyroid drugs in 77 pregnancies. Br. J. Obstet. Gynaecol. 87:970, 1980.

Smith SCH, Bold AM: Interpretation of in-vitro thyroid function tests during pregnancy. Br. J. Obstet. Gynaecol. 90:532, 1983.

Ramsay I, Kaaur S, Krassas G: Thyrotoxicosis in pregnancy: Results of treatment by antithyroid drugs combined with T4. Clin. Endocrinol. 18:73, 1983.

Pekonen F, Teramo K, Ikonen E, et al: Women on thyroid hormone therapy: Pregnancy course, fetal outcome, and amniotic fluid thyroid hormone level. Obstet. Gynecol. 63:635, 1984.

Thomas R, Reid R: Thyroid disease and reproductive dysfunction: A review. Obstet. Gynecol. 70:789, 1987.

Collagen Vascular Disease

Mor-Yosef S, Navot D, Rabinowitz R, et al: Collagen diseases in pregnancy. Obstet. Gynecol Surv. 39:67, 1984.

Lockshin MD, Druzin ML, Goei S, et al: Antibody to cardiolipin as a predictor of fetal distress or death in pregnant patients with systemic lupus erythematosus. N. Engl. J. Med. 313:152, 1985.

Lubbe WF, Liggins GC: Lupus anticoagulant and pregnancy.   Am. J. Obstet. Gynecol. 153:322, 1985.

Mintz G, Niz J, Gutierrez G, et al: Prospective study of pregnancy in systemic lupus erythematosus. Results of a multidisciplinary approach. J. Rheumatol. 13:732, 1986.

Urowitz M, Gladman D: Rheumatic disease in pregnancy. In Medical Complications during Pregnancy, edited by GN Burrow, T Ferris, ed. 3. Philadelphia, W.B. Saunders, 1988, pp 499-525.

Asthma

Hernandez E, Angell CS, Johnson JWC: Asthma in pregnancy: Current concepts. Obstet. Gynecol. 55:739, 1980.

de Swiet M: Maternal pulmonary disorders. In Maternal-Fetal Medicine Principles and Practice, edited by R. Creasy, R. Resnik.   Philadelphia, Saunders, 1984, pp 781-794.

Greenberger PA, Patterson R: Management of asthma during pregnancy. N. Engl. J. Med. 312:897, 1985.

Drugs for asthma.   Med. Letter 29, January, 30, 1987.

Weinberger S, Weiss S: Pulmonary Diseases in Medical Complications during Pregnancy, edited by GN Burrow, T Ferris, ed. 3.   Philadelphia, W.B. Saunders, 1988, pp 448-484.

Inflammatory Bowel Disease

Willoughby CP, Truelove SC: Ulcerative colitis and pregnancy.   Gut. 21:469, 1980.

Mogadam M, Dobbins WO, Korelitz BI, et al: Pregnancy in inflammatory bowel disease: Effect of sulfasalazine and corticosteroids on fetal outcome. Gastroenterol. 80:72, 1981.

Vender RJ, Spiro HM: Inflammatory bowel disease and pregnancy.   J. Clin. Gastroenterol. 4:231, 1982.

Sorokin JJ, Levine SM: Pregnancy and inflammatory bowel disease: A review of the literature.   Obstet. Gynecol. 62:247, 1983.

Connon J: Gastrointestinal complications. In Medical Complications during Pregnancy, edited by GN Burrow, T Ferris, ed. 3.   Philadelphia, W.B. Saunders, 1988, pp 303-317.

Chapter 3

Antepartum Obstetric Complications

First Trimester Bleeding

Approximately one-fourth of all pregnant patients will have some vaginal bleeding in early pregnancy. Along with a threatened or incomplete abortion, other causes include incorrect menstrual dating, lesion of the cervix, ectopic pregnancy, missed abortion, and trophoblastic disease. A systematic examination is necessary to search for any abdominal tenderness, internal cervical os dilation, uterine enlargement, and an adnexal mass. A proposed management plan is shown on the following page. Ultrasound scanning is of greater value than hormone assays in our experience. The prognosis is favorable if fetal motion is seen in utero beyond 6 weeks gestation.

Abnormal Pap Smear

Pregnancy may contribute to an increased incidence of abnormal **pap** smears because of cervical eversion. However, a worsening of abnormal cytologic findings is not thought to occur, and many **pap** smear abnormalities improve after delivery. Carcinoma in situ of the cervix is found in 1 in every 761 pregnant women, while invasive cervical carcinoma occurs in 1 in 2,200 pregnancies. A **pap** smear should be obtained routinely during the pelvic exam at the initial prenatal visit.

The widespread availability of colposcopy has dramatically reduced the frequency of conization to manage this problem. Mild dysplasia or inflammatory changes are best left untreated, with a **pap** smear being obtained later in gestation. The proposed management algorithm on the following page is recommended for evaluating the pregnant patient with moderate dysplasia or more advanced cellular atypia. Endocervical curettage is not performed routinely during pregnancy because of bleeding and ascending infection hazards. Biopsies of very suspicious areas may be performed, but capability for adequate hemostasis (ex. application of silver nitrate) is necessary. Conizations are rarely

Proposed Management for First Trimester Bleeding

Clinical suspicion
Vaginal bleeding confirmation
Cervix closed (if open internal os: inevitable or
 incomplete abortion)
Lower abdominal tenderness and/or adnexal mass

Hemodynamically unstable — Hemodynamically stable

Rapid fluid resuscitation

Ultrasound scan
Serum hCG (radioreceptor
 assay)

Operative intervention

+ hCG,
"Snowstorm"
on scan

+ hCG,
gestational
sac (intra-
uterine pregnancy
confirmed)

+ hCG,
no gesta-
tional sac

- hCG,
no gestational
sac (nonpregnant;
menstrual
irregularity)

More than   Less than
5 weeks   5 weeks

Consider
curettage

Quantitative hCG,
suction curettage
(trophoblastic disease)

Laparoscopy;   Either
possible   observation,
laparotomy   with culdocentesis
(R/O ectopic   or possible
pregnancy)   laparoscopy depending
                    on severity of
                    clinical symptoms and
                    degree of suspicion

Fetal limb   No fetal limb or
and heart   heart activity
activity

Observe   D & C if beyond
(threatened   8 weeks (slight
abortion)   ovum or missed
Repeat   abortion)
ultrasound if
bleeding persists

Proposed Management for an Abnormal Pap Smear in Pregnancy

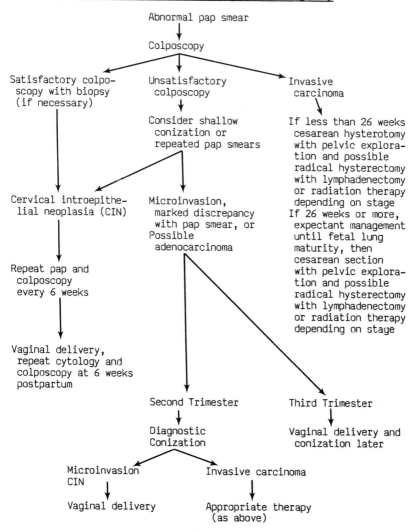

necessary. Regardless of the mode of therapy, pregnancy is not thought to affect long-term survival.

Rh Isoimmunization

In the last two decades the widespread use of Rh immune globulin (RhoGAM) has diminished remarkably the incidence of Rh isoimmunization. It remains a potentially serious complication of pregnancy, and a successful perinatal outcome requires careful planning during the antepartum, intrapartum, and neonatal periods. Along with a knowledge of the maternal serum antibody titer to the specific erythrocyte antigen, the gestational age, father's blood type and Rh antigen status must be determined. Most cases involve sensitization (formation of IgG antibodies) to the D, C, d, c, E and Kell blood groups. There is no need for further evaluation if the father is known to also be negative for that particular antigen. Hemolytic disease associated with certain less common and atypical antigens may be variable in severity (Table 3.1).

The level of maternal antibody titer is usually predictive of the severity of fetal disease in the first sensitized pregnancy. The antibody titer is of less prognostic value in subsequent pregnancies. Inutero transfusion or preterm delivery are becoming less common and should not be performed on the basis of an antibody titer alone. Instead, an amniotic fluid delta OD_{450} analysis is more predictive of fetal status and a fetal hematocrit determined by cordcentesis (needle inserted into umbilical vein for blood sampling or transfusion) is even more so. This technique is relatively new, at the stage of applied research, and not currently available at all institutions. It allows for direct evaluation of fetal hematologic status, and eliminates some falsely elevated delta OD_{450} results caused by old blood or meconium in the amniotic fluid.

Delivery should always be planned carefully. The standard means for assessing fetal well-being should be used. Particular attention should be placed on any decrease in fetal activity. Lung maturation is neither delayed nor accelerated in the isoimmunized pregnancy. Communication with blood bank and neonatal personnel is required to support the severely ill premature fetus and to prevent long-term neonatal complications.

Management of Atypical Antibody Screen

If the patient's antibody titer is below the "critical titer" established by that particular laboratory (usually 1:16 or less), it should be repeated at 20 weeks and then monthly. Provided the titer remains below the critical level, no intervention is necessary, and delivery at term can be anticipated.

Table 3.1
Examples of Antibodies Causing Hemolytic Disease

Blood Group System	Antigens Related to Hemolytic Disease	Severity of Hemolytic Disease
Rh	c	Mild to severe
	C	Mild to moderate
	D	Mild to severe
	e	Mild to moderate
	E	Mild to severe
Lewis		Not a proved cause of hemolytic disease of the newborn
I		Not a proved cause of hemolytic disease of the newborn
Kell	K	Mild to severe with hydrops fetalis
	k	Mild to severe
Duffy	Fy^a	Mild to severe with hydrops fetalis
	Fy^b	Not a cause of hemolytic disease
Kidd	Jk^a	Mild to severe
	Jk^b	Mild to severe
MNSs	M	Mild to severe
	N	Mild
	S	Mild to severe
	s	Mild to severe
Lutheran	Lu^a	Mild
	Lu^b	Mild
Diego	Di^a	Mild to severe
	Di^b	Mild to severe
Xg	Xg^a	Mild
P	$PP^1P^k(Tj^a)$	Mild to severe

Any patient with an initial antibody titer above the critical titer should have an amniocentesis or cordcentesis performed between 22-26 weeks or in the case of a rising titer as soon as it is recognized that the value has risen to exceed the critical titer.

Real-time ultrasonography is a necessary adjunct for evaluating fetal status. Signs of congestive heart failure would include pericardial effusion, scalp and scrotal edema, ascites, polyhydramnios, placental thickening (more than 5 cm), and diminished body motion. Ultrasonography is also helpful in guiding a 22-gauge needle for either an amniocentesis or cordcentesis.

When an amniocentesis is performed, it may be done as early as 22 weeks gestation for delta OD_{450} determination (indirectly measuring bilirubin concentration from hemolysis). We use a 22-gauge spinal needle and avoid insertion through the placenta. Results are plotted on the Liley curve shown in Figure 3.1.

The management outlined in the following flow chart is dependent on whether the delta OD_{450} value remains within zone 1, 2, or 3 on the

Evaluation after an Elevated Atypical Antibody

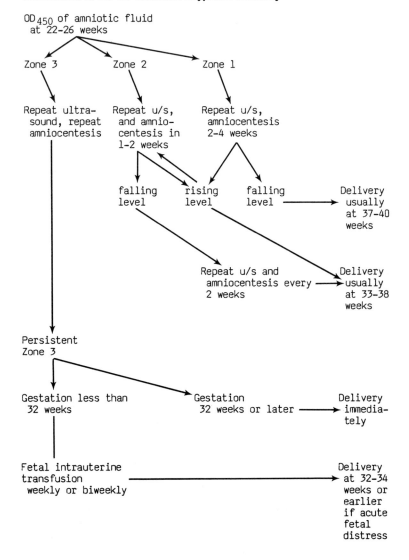

The management outlined in the following flow chart is dependent on whether the delta OD   value remains within zone 1, 2, or 3 on the Liley curve.   Fortunately the need for in utero transfusion is rare. Fetal transfusion by umbilical vein catheterization is beginning to replace intraabdominal transfusion at specialized perinatal centers. This technique, using ultrasound guidance, has allowed for a better assessment of the severity of fetal anemia and may delay further the need for premature delivery.   Before delivery of a severely affected infant, O negative blood or blood compatible with the mother's should be available for possible exchange transfusion by the pediatricians.   A direct Coomb's, hemoglobin, serum bilirubin, and blood type will need to be done on the newborn infant.

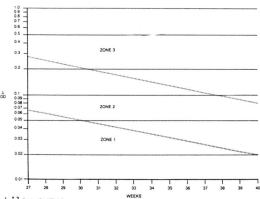

Figure 3.1.   Liley curve

Premature Labor

Approximately 7-10% of pregnant patients in the United States deliver prematurely.   These premature infants account for 75% of all perinatal mortality.   Most preliminary reports concerning prematurity prevention programs are positive.   While there is some conflicting data, and further studies are necessary, it is important for the obstetrician to be aware of conditions associated with premature labor (Table 3.2).   Bedrest and frequent cervical examinations are necessary.   Ambulatory uterine activity monitoring may be helpful especially in pregnancies complicated by prior premature labor deliveries, twins, or arrested premature labors.   In cases where contractions develop and continue despite the above measures, most patients will become candidates for tocolytic therapy.

While newer tocolytic drugs have been designed which decrease the incidence of side effects, these medications may cause significant alterations in maternal metabolism.   To prevent serious complications, the obstetrician must be aware of the proper selection criteria and safeguards required with the use of these agents.

Table 3.2
Conditions Associated with the Onset of Premature Labor

Maternal	Uterine
Acute severe systemic illness	Polyhydramnios
Chronic severe systemic illness	Foreign body (IUD)
Pyelonephritis, urinary tract	Trauma, surgical manipulation
infection	Cervical incompetence
Chronic hypertension	Uterine anomalies
Hyperthyroidism	Amniocentesis
Hyperparathyroidism	Abdominal surgery
Hyperadrenalism	Chorioamnionitis
Previous history of premature	Prior conization
labor	Fetoplacental
Fever or disseminated infection	Fetal death
Inadequate nutrition	Placenta previa
Age (under 16, over 40 years)	Abruptio placenta
Excess smoking	Fetal anomalies
Severe dehydration	Multifetal gestation
Abdominal trauma	Ruptured membranes
	Fetal growth retardation

Table 3.3
Contraindications to Tocolytic Therapy

Absolute	
Fetal death	Severe cardiac disease
Fetal congenital abnormality	Severe preeclampsia
incompatible with life	Active vaginal bleeding
Life threatening maternal	Unexplained uterine bleeding
illness	Chorioamnionitis

Relative	
Documented fetal pulmonary	Placenta previa with
maturity	minimal bleeding
Diabetes (beta-agonists)	Abruptio placenta
Mild cardiac disease	Preterm ruptured membranes
Pulmonary disease	Vascular headaches
Hypertensive disorders	

Before beginning drug therapy to inhibit uterine contractions, true labor must be accurately diagnosed and any accompanying obstetric or medical disorders should be sought. The criteria for selecting patients for tocolytic therapy is outlined below, and recommended pre-therapy screening tests are listed in Table 3.4.

Table 3.4
Tests before Beginning Tocolytic Therapy

Cervical cultures for gonorrhea, Group B beta-hemolytic strepto-
cocci, and chlamydia
Clean catch midsteam or catheterized urine specimen for
urinalysis and culture
Confirmation of the presence or absence of ruptured membranes
Ultrasound exam for BPD/femur length, fetal presentation, twins,
amniotic fluid volume, fetal anomaly, uterine anomaly, estimated
fetal weight, site for possible amniocentesis
Baseline fetal heart rate tracing
Complete blood count with differential
Serum electrolytes
Electrocardiogram (if maternal cardiac disease)

---

    a.   Clinical diagnosis
          Gestational age between 20 and 36 weeks
          Estimated fetal weight less than 2,500 gm (especially
          1,500 gm or less)
          Uterine contractions every 10 min or less, lasting
          30 sec or more, for at least a 30 min period
          Cervical dilation of 4 cm or less
    b.   No remarkable antepartum complication or contraindication
        (Table 3.3)

No group of tocolytic drugs has been definitely shown to be ideal
in inhibiting premature labor. Side effects from these drugs in the
mother and fetus must be recognized, and patient education is
necessary. Careful monitoring of the fetal heart rate and uterine
activity is paramount. When an undesired effect from a specific drug
is manifested, or when intravenous therapy is required for more than
24-48 hr, the drug may be continued, discontinued, reduced in dosage,
or a second drug used in combination. These decisions should be made
by the clinican based on an evaluation of the seriousness of the side
effect, the probability of premature delivery, and the potential
consequences of premature delivery at the current gestational age.

Drug Therapy

Ritodrine

    Ritodrine hydrochloride remains the only FDA approved tocolytic
drug. It is a selective beta-2 receptor agonist which acts primarily
by inhibiting smooth muscle uterine contractions. Beta-2 receptors may
also be found in the bronchioles and blood vessels, and their
stimulation results in bronchial relaxation and hypotension. Ritodrine
is also a weak beta-1 receptor agonist, and tachycardia is common.

Alpha-receptors are not usually stimulated using ritodrine, so hypertension is very uncommon.

An intravenous solution of ritodrine in 5% dextrose in water (150 mg/500 ml) is the standard concentration of drug in intravenous fluids. A loading dose is unnecessary and maintenance therapy consists of an initial infusion of 100 mcg/min (20 ml/hr) with upward dose adjustments in 50 mcg/min increments to a maximum level of 350 mcg/min (70 ml/hr). Maintenance therapy is titrated according to contraction frequency and may be continued for several days if necessary. It is usually continued for 12 hrs after the arrest of labor before the patient is begun on oral therapy.

Oral therapy is usually started an hour before discontinuing the intravenous regimen and is begun once uterine contractions are barely palpable. Oral therapy consists of 10 mg every 2 hrs initially. The dose is then titrated to maintain a maternal pulse of 90-100 and the absence of contractions. It usually ranges from 10-20 mg every 2-6 hrs. Only rarely should the oral dose exceed 120 mg/day.

If labor recurs, the patient should be reexamined carefully. The infusion may be restarted if no contraindications to tocolysis are found. The initial ritodrine infusion will inadequately inhibit labor in approximately 50% of patients. These patients are at high risk for subclinical intrauterine infection, and amniocentesis for gram stain and culture and sensitivity may be appropriate. The addition of a simultaneous magnesium sulfate infusion, as outlined below, will result in the successful treatment of half of these patients. However, if labor persists or once fetal pulmonary maturity has developed, the medications should be discontinued.

The most frequent side effects with intravenous ritodrine are cardiovascular. The maternal heart rate may increase up to 40 beats/min above the baseline, and the pulse pressure may widen up to 20 mm Hg as the intravenous dose is increased. If this results in troublesome symptoms relief can often be obtained by reducing the dose for a short period of time. Later it can usually be increased again without recurrence of symptoms. Pulmonary edema has been reported in patients who are also receiving glucocorticoids or excessive intravenous fluids. Hypotonic solutions or 5% dextrose in water should be used.

Transient metabolic problems may include hyperglycemia, hyperinsulinemia, lipemia, ketonemia, hyperlacticacidemia, and hypokalemia. Unpleasant side effects may include tremor (10-15%), restlessness (20%), and palpitations (33%). Other beta-agonists (terbutaline, isoxsuprine) may be used as alternatives if these symptoms persist.

It may be helpful to determine a serum potassium before initiating intravenous therapy, and any history of cardiac disease or chest tightness requires a baseline electrocardiogram. Hypotension may be avoided with the patient remaining in a lateral recumbent position during intravenous therapy.

Neonatal complications may include bradycardia, hypotension, and hypoglycemia.

Magnesium Sulfate

Magnesium sulfate is useful in inhibiting premature uterine contractions using doses which are approximately twice those used for seizure prophylaxis in preeclamptic patients. This drug may also be used in combination with ritodrine, so that uterine contractions may be inhibited more effectively or when unwanted side effects from ritodrine therapy require smaller doses to be administered.

A 40 gm dose of magnesium sulfate is mixed in 1 liter of 5% dextrose in water or 0.45 normal saline. The loading dose is usually 4 gm in 100 ml over 20 min followed by maintenance therapy of 1-4 gm/hr intravenously. After successful intravenous therapy, oral ritodrine may be initiated. Oral magnesium gluconate in a dose of 1 mg every 4 hrs may be employed if there is a contraindication, failure, or intolerable side effects from oral beta-agonist therapy.

A baseline serum magnesium level may be useful, and signs of hypermagnesemia (hyporeflexia, depressed respiratory rate) should be sought periodically.

Respiratory depression in the neonate is very uncommon from in utero magnesium exposure but can occur in low birthweight infants with decreased urine output.

Terbutaline

Although not FDA approved for this indiction, terbutaline is another beta-agonist which has been used in place of ritodrine in many highly respected institutions. Their mechanisms of action and side effects are similar. While some investigators have claimed greater efficacy and fewer complications in comparison to ritodrine, their observations are questioned by other authorities due to lack of information regarding equipotent dosages. The major advantage of terbutaline would appear to be its considerably lower cost. For intravenous therapy, a 20 mcg/ml solution is infused beginning at a rate of 2.5 mcg/min (0.125 ml/min) and increased by 2.5 mcg/min at 20 min intervals until labor is stopped, unacceptable cardiovascular side effects occur, or a maximum dose of 17.5 mcg/min (0.875 ml/min) is reached. The oral dosage is approximately 5 mg every 4 hrs but should be titrated to the maternal pulse and uterine contraction frequency as for ritodrine.

Indomethacin

This prostaglandin inhibitor has been shown to successfully arrest premature labor. There is concern that prolonged use may result in a narrowing or premature closure of the ductus arteriosus and a persistent fetal circulation. Short term therapy (less than 72 hrs) may occasionally be helpful to allow for steroid treatment to enhance fetal pulmonary maturity in patients refractory to more traditional tocolytics. A 25 mg dose may be given orally or rectally every 4-6 hrs.

Neonatal Survival Rates

When premature delivery is anticipated, it is necessary to counsel the patient about the chances that the baby will survive in the intensive care nursery and be discharged home. Listed in Table 3.5 are survival percentages according to gestational age and birthweight for inborn infants admitted to the University of Nebraska Intensive Care Nursery between 1981 and 1986. The data exclude infants with life-threatening anomalies. It is appropriate for each institution to develop its own survival statistics in order to make sound therapeutic judgments and to counsel patients adequately.

Table 3.5
Neonatal Survival Rates at the University of Nebraska Medical Center According to Gestational Age and Birth Weight (1981-1987)*

Gestational Age (weeks)	% Survivors	Birth Weight (gm)	% Survivors
24	0	500	0
25	22	501-800	22
26	48	800-1,000	75
27	75	1,001-1,250	82
28	83	1,251-1,500	94
29	94	1,501-1,750	97
30	95	1,751-2,500	98
31	95	> 2,500	99
32	97		
> 33	99		

*These rates are for singleton infants without life-threatening anomalies. Survival rates may be slightly lower for multifetal gestations delivered before 30 weeks.

Preterm Rupture of Membranes

Premature rupture of the membranes (PROM) is defined as spontaneous rupture of the amniotic membranes (amniorexis) occurring at any gestational age before the onset of labor. A latent period usually lasts at least one hour. The incidence of PROM ranges from 4.5-7.6% of all pregnancies. Preterm PROM occurs in approximately 1% of pregnancies and clearly represents a more pressing problem for the obstetrician.

Diagnosis

Diagnosis requires visualization of amniotic fluid leaking from the cervical os or in the vaginal vault, testing any fluid for a basic pH (nitrazine positivity), and ferning. This should be accomplished during sterile speculum examination. Cervical cultures for Group B beta-streptococci and gonorrhea (in certain populations) should be obtained, prolapsed cord ruled out, and cervical effacement and dilitation estimated during this initial examination. The subsequent development of infection has been highly correlated with the interval (hours) from initial digital examination. Therefore, digital examination should be avoided unless the patient is clearly in labor and/or a decision has been made to effect delivery. Ultrasound may be useful to document the gestational age, estimated fetal weight, decreased amniotic fluid, fetal presentation, twins, and any fetal malformation. If the diagnosis of PROM still remains in doubt, the instillation of 3-5 ml of sterile fluorescein ophthalmologic solution by amniocentesis, followed by inspection of the vagina under black light illumination for the characteristic fluorescent pattern will usually resolve the issue.

Management

General Measures

The obstetrician is required to balance the relative risks of prematurity and infection. These risks may vary from population to population and at various gestational ages. When possible, local data should be considered in formulating an institution's management protocols. Discussion with the neonatal staff is essential and maternal transfer to a tertiary care center is urged if a septic premature infant is anticipated. However, it is appropriate to remain cognizant of certain general principles.

Dating is often very difficult after the occurrence of PROM. The resultant oligohydramnios may depress fundal height, and impair ultrasonic evaluation. Biparietal diameters and abdominal circumferences may be falsely lowered, but femur length measurements are usually relatively reliable.

Fetal distress, particularly cord compression, is much more common than in idiopathic premature labor. This is especially true if the fetus has a precarious lie (breech, back up transverse). In those patients whose fetuses have achieved potentially viable gestational age, initial evaluation should include a prolonged period of electronic fetal monitoring. Subsequently, the gravida should be instructed in daily fetal movement charting, since fetal activity is not impaired with PROM. Prolonged nonstress tests or biophysical profiles should be performed at 24-48 hr intervals. When labor develops, prophylactic amniotransfusion may be undertaken, since it is associated with a marked reduction in the frequency and severity of abnormal fetal heart rate patterns. An intrauterine pressure catheter is introduced, and normal saline infused through a blood warming coil attached to the catheter at a rate of 10 ml/min for the first hour and then at a rate of 3 ml/min.

Surveillance is required to detect potential chorioamnionitis. Maternal temperature should be recorded at least every 4 hours. The presence of an elevated white blood count may provide confirmatory evidence of clinically suspected infection, but it has been demonstrated repeatedly not to offer any enhanced predictive value over clinical signs. Therefore, the expense of daily blood count monitoring does not appear justified. C-reactive protein may provide further laboratory evidence of infection in the presence of an elevated leukocyte count. Amniocentesis for gram stain, culture and sensitiviity can be accomplished in approximately 50-60% of women with PROM. The presence of bacteria on gram stain of unspun amniotic fluid (or a subsequent positive culture) is associated with clinical evidence of maternal or neonatal infection in 50-60% of patients. Other investigators have reported a persistently decreased amniotic fluid volume, a nonreactive nonstress test, or an abnormal biophysical profile to have equal or better predictive accuracy for infection in this population.

Patients with PROM frequently demonstrate fetal pulmonary maturity at relatively early gestational ages. If free-flowing fluid can be obtained from the vaginal vault, the L/S ratio is usually quite similar to that obtained by amniocentesis, and if phosphatidylglycerol is present, it is always present at amniocentesis. When vaginal fluid cannot be obtained, an amniocentesis should be considered.

Most randomized studies have shown little or no benefit to result from the use of either intravenous tocolytics or corticosteroids (for the enhancement of fetal pulmonary maturity) in pregnancies complicated by PROM. Most obstetric authorities do not recommend the use of these medications in this condition.

At Term

Ninety percent of these patients will enter spontaneous labor within 24 hrs, and present few management problems. Several studies have demonstrated increased perinatal mortality, when the latent period exceeds 24 hrs. We usually follow a policy of inducing or augmenting labor as necessary to achieve delivery within this time interval. On the other hand, aggressive attempts to induce gravidas with long and closed cervices (unfavorable Bishop scores) are associated with higher rates of operative delivery. Therefore, expectant management is necessary with careful evaluation for infection and fetal distress.

33-37 weeks

In this group of patients, the risk of neonatal hyaline membrane disease is very low when 16 hrs or longer have elapsed since the membranes have ruptured. We utilize oxytocin induction in most instances to attempt to accomplish delivery shortly after 16 hrs. If the Bishop score is extremely unfavorable, conservative management is acceptable.

24-32 weeks

The risk of pulmonary immaturity outweighs the risk of infection in this subpopulation. Conservative measures according to the principles outlined above are practiced in most tertiary centers. The patient should be advised that even with conservative therapy approximately 50% of patients will begin labor within 24 hrs and 75% within 5 days.

Before 24 weeks

Any patient with well documented PROM before the 24th gestational week should be informed that the probability of leaving the hospital with a living normal child is very poor, perhaps as low as 25%. Many of these children develop pulmonary hypoplasia and/or orthopedic deformities, die in utero, or deliver at very early gestational ages. The option of pregnancy termination should be discussed. The patient may elect conservative therapy in the hope that the fetus will grow and mature despite the unfavorable odds.

Corticosteroids to Enhance Fetal Lung Maturity

The use of corticosteroids to accelerate fetal pulmonary maturity remains a controversial topic in obstetrics. Most studies involving the use of betamethasone, hydrocortisone, or dexamethasone have revealed significant reductions in incidences of respiratory distress and neonatal deaths when corticosteriods have been given before anticipated delivery, especially betweeen 28-32 weeks. Developmental evaluation of treated fetuses who are now school age children have not revealed any adverse effects with such short-term therapy.

Indications

The anticipated delivery of a premature infant requires a prompt and accurate evaluation of fetal pulmonary maturity by amniotic fluid testing if possible. An L/S ratio of less than 2:1 or the absence of phosphatidylglycerol suggests fetal lung immaturity. A trial of corticosteroid therapy may be useful in enhancing fetal lung maturity, especially between the 24th and 32nd weeks of gestation.

When fetal lung maturity testing is not readily available (such as at night, or weekends, and during holidays), corticosteroid therapy may be administered empirically if the gestational age is 32 weeks or less and impending delivery is anticipated. Good clinical judgement is necessary, realizing that a time lapse must exist between maternal treatment and a fetal response. The underlying antepartum complication should be expected to remain stabilized; otherwise, delivery should take place regardless of any corticosteroid therapy.

General Considerations

Although there is controversy in the pediatric literature, corticosteroid treatment does not appear to be helpful for pregnancies complicated by preterm rupture of the amniotic membranes. Most investigators conclude that there is no association between maternal and neonatal infection with the use of short-term corticosteroid therapy, however. Any advantage to this therapy in addition to conservative management alone remains unclear. Corticosteroids may increase the white blood count (primarily neutrophils), so clinical criteria and appropriate cultures are especially important to screen for infection.

Hypertension is not thought to be exacerbated, and fetal mortality is not considered to be increased with steroid therapy. Nevertheless, pregnancy intervention is necessary during such therapy when hypertension worsens.

Corticosteroids may accentuate glucose intolerance because of the increased insulin requirements occurring from the inhibition of glucose utilization, mobilization of amnio acids for conversion to glucose and glycogen, and induction of liver enzymes for gluconeogenesis. Steroid therapy is therefore not recommended when preterm delivery of the severe diabetic is anticipated.

Patients whose pregnancy is complicated by a multifetal gestation should receive the same dose of steroids as is given in singleton pregnancies, however less enhancement of fetal lung maturity may ultimately result.

Fetal sex determination by ultrasound visualization before amniocentesis for fetal lung maturity may be useful in predicting which pregnancies would benefit from therapy. Antenatally administered corticosteroids may be more helpful in promoting fetal lung maturity in female rather than male fetuses. We do prescribe this medication even if the fetus is a male, but do explain this limitation to the parents.

Prompt delivery is necessary in the presence of severe vaginal bleeding. Minimal bleeding such as that found with a placenta previa may permit conservative therapy and glucocorticoid treatment. Drug therapy may be initiated once any excessive bleeding has subsided and a normal platelet count has been obtained.

Contraindications to Therapy

Fortunately, absolute contraindications to corticosteroid therapy are uncommon. Maternal contraindications include tuberculosis, active herpes, or febrile illness or other infections. Corticosteroid therapy is also contraindicated in the presence of amnionitis, imminent delivery, a mature amniotic fluid test result, or an inability to monitor the fetus.

Steroids may be given with caution in those pregnancies complicated by borderline hypertension, well-controlled diabetes mellitus, hyperthyroidism, placental insufficiency, minimal uterine bleeding, or premature labor adequately treated with beta-agonists or magnesium sulfate.

Drug Choice and Dose Regimen

The best specific drug and appropriate dosage are presently unknown. Neither hydrocortisone, dexamethasone, or betamethasone has been clearly shown to offer advantages in promoting fetal lung maturity, although betamethasone is the drug used most commonly at most university medical centers. All of the above rapidly cross the placenta. Drug dose regimens used to enhance fetal lung maturation are shown in Table 3.6. A treatment regimen using the least effective dose for the shortest duration has not been established.

The shortest period for the drug to be effective is believed to be 24 hrs after the final dose. If 7 or more days have elapsed after completing the drug therapy, repeat amniotic fluid testing (with an L/S less than 2 or negative pG) is preferred before prescribing another course of therapy.

Table 3.6
Corticosteroid Dosage Regimens

Drug	Dosage Schedule	Total Dose
Betamethasone	12 mg IM q 12-24 hr for 2 doses	24 mg
Dexamethasone	4 mg IM q 8 hr for 6 doses	24 mg
Hydrocortisone	500 mg IV q 8 hr for 4 doses	2 gm

Multifetal Gestation

Although a twin gestation is reportedly found in 1 in 80 pregnancies, the actual incidence is higher as more multifetal gestations which may abort are diagnosed by ultrasonography in early gestation. Early diagnosis and careful management are necessary for optimal care, since virtually every medical and obstetric complication associated with pregnancy is more common in a multifetal gestation.

Antepartum Management

A high index of suspicion is necessary for early diagnosis. Clues would include the following: elderly multigravida, maternal family history of dizygotic twins, fertility pills (clomiphene: 6% twinning, pergonal: 25% twinning) uterine size greater than menstrual dates (as early as end of first trimester), and presenting fetal part smaller than anticipated. Proper care requires frequent clinic visits (check cervix, blood pressure, Hct, diabetes screen, etc.), serial ultrasound exams (approximately every 4-6 weeks), and proper nutrition (folate and iron supplementation; 300 additional calories per day, avoid excess salt).

A cervical cerclage for twinning alone is not justified. Guidelines for tocolytic drugs and corticosteroid therapy for the singleton fetus are applicable to the multifetal gestation. Half of twins are born before 34 weeks, so frequent cervical examination, additional daily rest periods, and perhaps ambulatory uterine activity monitoring are justified to prevent premature labor.

Supportive care and patient education are necessary. Discussions should include pain relief during labor, potential complications before or during labor, and care of the infants after delivery. The babies' doctor should be aware of the pregnancy and informed during labor.

In the event of a preterm fetal demise, immediate delivery is not advisable unless late in gestation. A twin-twin transfusion should be suspected, and delivery should be considered if 28 weeks or beyond. Maternal serum fibrinogen levels should be drawn weekly to search for any coagulopathy. Obstructed labor is possible.

Amniotic fluid retrieved from only one gestational sac is usually all that is necessary for fetal lung maturity testing. The sac containing the "healthier" of the two fetuses should be sampled. Criteria for interpreting fetal lung tests is the same as for singleton pregnancies.

The performance and interpretation of many fetal surveillance techniques are limited with multifetal gestations. As a general rule, if the mother is healthy and if fetal growth is appropriate (by clinical exam and ultrasonography), no further testing is necessary. The same principles for nonstress testing, biophysical profile assessment, and fetal movement charting in the singleton fetus apply for the multifetal gestation. Periodic ultrasound examination is the most useful means for assessing fetal growth and well-being. Ultrasound may also be useful in locating the placenta, conjoined twins, or any space-occupying anomalies.

Intrapartum Management

The anesthesia, neonatal, and obstetric staff should be notified when the patient is admitted to the labor floor. The patient should be typed and crossmatched for possible transfusion. If time permits, a bedside real-time ultrasound examination should be performed to search for: two separate sacs, a major anomaly (including conjoined twins), fetal presentations, fetal growth disparity, and placental localization, especially if a cesarean section is planned.

Cesarean Section
1.   Suggested indications:
               Twin A: breech
               Fetal distress
               Prolapsed cord
               Three or more fetuses
               Delivery before 33 weeks or fetal weights 1,500 gm or less

Delivery of twin B if fetal distress, prolapsed cord, constricted uterine ring (despite halothane), persistent abnormal presentation, or twin B larger with failure to descend adequately
2. Prophylactic antibiotics are indicated
3. Occasionally vertical skin and uterine incisions for adequate space
4. Epidural anesthesia preferable with uterus displaced off inferior vena cava.

Vaginal Delivery
1. Labor on left side
2. Supplemental oxygen
3. Electronic monitoring of fetal heart rate and uterine contractions
   a. Fetal heart rate: internal electrode - Twin A, external transducer - Twin B
   b. Uterine contractions: internal uterine catheter connected in series to both monitors
4. No regional anesthesia until cervical dilation 4 cm or more. May use intravenous narcotic sparingly or nitrous oxide by controlled face mask
5. If uterine inertia exists, oxytocin may be used
6. Two obstetricians (including staff) in attendance at delivery
7. Large episiotomy
8. Twin A delivered in the usual manner as a singleton
9. No absolute time for delivery of second twin as long as monitoring fetal heart rate and watching for any excess hemorrhage (possible abruption). Ultrasonic visualization of the second twin may be performed in the delivery room to observe the fetal heart (rate and position) and to watch the examiner's hand during any extraction procedure.
10. May need halothane to relax uterus to guide the second twin into the pelvis and for partial breech extraction
11. If the second twin is breech, external version may be accomplished using ultrasound guidance after vaginal delivery of the first twin.

Postpartum Care

1. The zygosity of multiple fetuses has assumed more importance with advances in of organ transplantation. Twins of opposite sex are almost always dizygotic. Examination of the placenta may also aid in identifying the zygosity. Infants are monozygotic if there is only one amnionic sac (a rare finding) or juxtaposed amnions not separated by chorion. Most infants are dizygotic if adjacent amnions are separated by chorion. Blood obtained from the umbilical cord may be used to determine differences in major blood groups which would indicate dizygosity. More complicated techniques such as extensive blood and tissue antigen typing of the twins and parents may also be done if these simple procedures fail to confirm zygosity.

2. Maternal conditions requiring close observation include excessive fatigue, depression, and hemorrhage (uterine atony, lacerations, retained placental fragments).

Third Trimester Bleeding

Vaginal bleeding at any time during pregnancy may result from cervical erosion, polyps and carcinoma, and trauma. The most common causes of third trimester bleeding include labor, placental abruption, or placenta previa. A vasa previa or uterine rupture should also be considered.

With the exception of labor or "show", these conditions are potentially life-threatening to the mother and fetus and frequently result in premature delivery. Successful management requires anticipation of potential complications, rapid intervention to reverse complications, and competent neonatal assistance.

A thorough history is necessary to determine the amount and character of the bleeding, any pain, prior bleeding, trauma, any uterine anomaly, and activity of the fetus. Evaluation of the patient requires careful monitoring of her vital signs. Along with a general physical examination, the uterus should be examined for tone and tenderness. A digital pelvic exam should be performed only after ultrasonography has ruled out placenta previa. Fetal heart activity should also be sought to rule out the possibility of an intrauterine demise. Along with evaluating for fetal viability, an overall assessment of any labor and the extent of hemorrhage are necessary.

Initial laboratory tests should include a Kleihauer-Betke test, urinalysis, and coagulation studies (PT, PTT, platelet count, fibrinogen, fibrin split products). Any pooled vaginal blood should be obtained to test for fetal blood. The observation of clot formation is often as valuable as more complex coagulation studies. The APT test and the Fetaldex test have been used to determine whether the blood is maternal in origin. The APT test involves the mixing of any vaginal blood with an equal part of 0.25% sodium hydroxide. The blood will turn to a light brown color if it is maternal in origin; otherwise, it is of fetal origin. If the APT test result is not conclusive and bleeding persists, a Fetaldex test may be performed.

Depending on the extent of hemorrhage, an infusion of 5% glucose in Lactated Ringers solution is indicated using an 18-gauge or greater catheter. Continuous external fetal heart rate monitoring is required to search for any fetal tachycardia, loss of beat-to-beat variability or pathologic change. Two to four units of blood should be typed and crossmatched.

Ultrasonography should be performed as soon as possible. The diagnosis of a placenta previa may be made using ultrasonography, preferable to other x-ray techniques which are no longer used (soft tissue x-ray, isotope scans, amniography). Elevating the presenting fetal part transabdominally may permit a better view of the placenta in the lower pelvis. A placental abruption may appear as a sonolucent retroplacental mass or an elevation of the membranes on the contralateral side of the uterus which may expand or contract over time depending on the extent of hemorrhage and whether or not it is occult. Often the ultrasound examination is of no value if hemorrhage has occurred externally, since the sonolucent area is smaller in size and the retroplacental blood is homogenous with the placenta. During ultrasonic examination, it is also possible to search for fetal malformations, multifetal gestation, and fetal presentation. If expectant management is undertaken, serial ultrasound examinations should be performed to assess fetal growth and well-being.

Depending on the circumstance, an amniocentesis should be done for fetal lung maturity testing. Blood within the amniotic fluid suggests the diagnosis of an abruption. It also renders the L/S ratio less reliable. Testing for phosphatidyglycerol (PG) in addition to the L/S ratio is often necessary. However, the L/S ratio of blood is approximately 1.8/1.0, and levels above this value are usually reliable.

Tocolytic agents such as ritodrine should be used with caution. The diagnosis should be fairly certain, fetal distress should not be evident, and vaginal bleeding should not be sufficient to cause maternal hypotension.

If the pregnancy is not near term and there is no further bleeding while in the hospital, the patient may be discharged with proper precautions. She should usually be within a 30-min drive, and transportation should be readily available. The patient should be instructed on proper nutrition and discontinue any smoking. Physical activities should be restricted, and douching and sexual intercourse are contraindicated. She should be seen weekly on a outpatient basis, and a hematocrit should be drawn periodically. We recommend blood transfusion if the hematocrit is less than 30%. The telephone number of the clinic and labor hall should be given to the patient.

A double-setup examination is appropriate to rule out a placenta previa if the diagnosis remains questionable and the perinatal team is ready to commit the patient to delivery. This pelvic examination should be done in the operating room with preparations for cesarean section already being available.

Placenta Previa

"Silent" placenta previas are being diagnosed early in gestation with more frequent ordering of ultrasound examinations. Up to half of all placentas are either low lying or cover the cervical os in the second trimester, but only 2-3% of all placentas will remain within the lower uterine segment at term. This occurs most frequently in those patients whose placentas are central or complete in the second trimester.

Delivery by cesarean section is generally recommended if a placenta previa is apparent in a patient at 38 weeks or greater (or earlier with evidence of fetal lung maturity). A vaginal delivery with a very marginal placenta is possible but requires a double-setup examination and very close fetal and uterine monitoring.

In the absence of life threatening hemorrhage, approximately half of patients with a placenta previa remote from term may be treated with conservative therapy. Blood should be replaced and fetal-maternal monitoring initiated as outlined above. The patient usually requires hospitalization for 5 days or more. If bleeding persists, as evidenced by continuous spotting on the perineal pad, she should remain in the hospital with close fetal monitoring. If bleeding subsides, the patient may ambulate gradually. She may be discharged from the hospital once bleeding subsides if there is no evidence of fetal distress, especially if this is her first episode of bleeding.

More specific criteria for outpatient management of a pregnancy with a placenta previa include: 1) no active bleeding, 2) no anemia (Hct 35% or greater), 3) premature fetus, 4) patient lives within 30 min of hospital, 5) patient and relatives understand condition, and 6) telephone at home and reliable transportation. The precautions listed about proper nutrition and restrictions in physical activity would apply. The patient should be instructed on daily fetal movement charting and notifying her physician at once if there is any further bleeding, premature labor, fetal inactivity, or fever. While this management protocol has yielded excellent results on our services, other investigators have recently suggested that gestation is prolonged with continuous hospitalization until near term. Also, because neonatal intensive care costs were reduced substantially, inpatient care was more cost effective in the long run than outpatient management. Further studies will be required to substantiate or refute this finding.

A pelvic examination is to be performed only when a double set-up is undertaken. An ultrasound examination is useful for localizing the placenta before a cesarean section. If surgery is necessary, a high transverse or a vertical uterine incision is recommended if the placenta previa sweeps anteriorly. Occasionally, a placenta previa is associated with a placenta invading into the uterus (accreta or percreta), and cesarean hysterectomy may be necessary to control bleeding. It is important to discuss this possibility with the patient when obtaining informed consent for cesarean section.

Placental Abruption

A clinically evident placental abruption occurs in approximately 0.5-1% of pregnancies. It is most commonly associated with conditions leading to chronic uteroplacental insufficiency such as hypertension. It is also found commonly to accomodate a marginal previa. An abruption severe enough to cause intrauterine fetal demise occurs in 1/500 pregnancies. This diagnosis is usually one of exclusion if a placenta previa is not visualized on ultrasound examination. Fetal monitoring is desirable using nonstress tests, biophysical profiles, and fetal movement charting although the true value of these tests for this disorder is uncertain and limited.

If bleeding is minimal, the preterm pregnancy may be managed expectantly. However, if the bleeding continues or there is evidence of fetal lung maturity, an attempt should be made to expedite delivery.

Liberal use of cesarean section is indicated especially when there is any suggestion of fetal distress, or hemorrhage severe enough to cause fetal or maternal death. However, approximately half of pregnancies may be managed successfully with vaginal delivery.

An attempt at vaginal delivery is possible, but prolonged labor should be avoided. Prompt and adequate replacement of maternal blood loss is paramount, regardless of the time interval to delivery. An amniotomy is recommended to search for blood in the amniotic fluid, to facilitate labor, and to decrease the risk of thromboplastin release into the maternal circulation. The use of forceps to decrease the second stage of labor should be considered unless the risk of trauma is too great a concern. Examination of the placenta is useful, although not always diagnostic, and the pathologist should be notified of the expected diagnosis.

A placental abruption is likely to recur in one-tenth to one-fourth of subsequent pregnancies. The actual risk is dependent on associated medical or obstetric complications.

Hemorrhagic Shock

Hemorrhagic shock may follow excessive bleeding from a placenta previa or placental abruption, ischemic necrosis to distant organs (especially the anterior pituitary and kidney), or may result from the delayed diagnosis and inadequate replacement of lost blood.

When suspected, the mother and fetus should be monitored carefully and delivered promptly. The mother's vital signs should be monitored and recorded on a flow sheet. Urine output should be maintained at 25 ml/hr or greater. A central line may be used with central venous pressure maintained in the range of 8-15 cm of water. If left ventricular function is considered abnormal, pulmonary artery pressures may be determined using a Swan-Ganz catheter. The pulmonary artery pressure should be maintained below 18 mm Hg.

Replacement of blood loss requires the infusion of packed rbc's (Hct 60-65%) and fresh frozen plasma (all factors except platelets), in addition to the rapid administration of a 5% glucose and normal saline or Lactated Ringer's solution. A plasma expander such as albumin may also be administered to increase the intravascular volume. Heparin is not useful in treating the patient with hemorrhagic shock. Serum electrolytes, calcium, and arterial blood gases should be determined frequently because of potential fluid, electrolyte, and acid/base imbalances.

Postpartum Care

Most pregnant patients with third trimester bleeding will do satisfactorily after delivery. Any coagulation difficulties usually correct themselves within a short period.

Incisions should be inspected periodically for hematoma formation. Careful monitoring of the fluid intake and output is necessary to avoid hypo- or hypervolemia. The patient's blood count, electrolytes, and urine volume should be monitored closely within the first few days after delivery, and any imbalances should be corrected.

Infections of the genital tract are more common in patients who had profuse intrapartum vaginal bleeding. If prophylactic antibiotics have not been started, the patient should be monitored carefully for any endometritis or incisional infections.

Postdates

Between 2 and 11% of all pregnancies will remain undelivered for 2 weeks or more beyond the estimated date of confinement. This complication of pregnancy represents one of the most frequent abnormalities in routine obstetric care and is a common indicator for fetal well-being testing and induction of labor. The placenta is thought to degenerate with gestation advancing beyond the 37th week.

Perinatal morbidity and mortality increases beyond term, and the subsequent development of unborn infants may be compromised from impaired uteroplacental function. Most infants born to mothers with postdate pregnancies (42 weeks or more) do well, but distress in the fetus later found to be postmature is often not anticipated until after the onset of labor or shortly before delivery.

Most clinicians would agree that unless the cervix is favorable or an obstetric or medical complication is present, expectant or conservative management with frequent antepartum monitoring of the mother and fetus is preferable to routine intervention of the postdate pregnancy. This trend toward conservative management has been attributed to refinement in fetal surveillance testing. The incidence of an antepartum and intrapartum stillbirth has thus decreased significantly.

Perinatal morbidity in postdate pregnancies remains a major concern, however. Immediate problems in the newborn include asphyxia, meconium aspiration, seizure disorders, metabolic imbalances, and respiratory difficulties. These problems are more common in infants who experienced uteroplacental insufficiency. In addition to these immediate concerns, the infants are thought to be at greater risk of subsequent delayed development, sleep disturbance, and severe illness during infancy.

Between 12-43% (approximately 20%) of patients with postdate pregnancies deliver infants with classic findings of dysmaturity or postmaturity. These infants have long lean bodies with characteristic skin changes (leather-like consistency, little subcutaneous fat, and desquamation of the skin). Much hair, meconium staining, longer fingernails, and an alert facial expression may also be seen. Although these infants are often heavier than average for a term pregnancy, these physical findings suggest a form of intrauterine growth retardation.

Postdate pregnancies complicated by fetal postmaturity would therefore benefit from immediate and well-monitored intervention and meticulous care of the infant. Realizing that these infants are found in a minority of the postdate pregnancies, pregnancy intervention is not routinely recommended. The mother should be aware of the need for close monitoring and the increased possibility of a cesarean section. However, a worthwhile means for predicting a postmature fetus and in screening for fetal distress would be helpful.

Antepartum Management

A prerequisite to proper management in these cases is precise pregnancy dating. Information about the last menstrual period, quickening, auscultation of fetal heart tones, serial uterine fundal height examinations, and ultrasound examination(s) is always useful. With accurate gestational dating and the pregnancy now 2 weeks beyond the estimated date of confinement, a search for other complications and an examination of the cervix are indicated. If there is any other complication (such as hypertension) or if the cervix is "ripe", intervention is recommended by induction of labor if the fetus is in a cephalic presentation.

If accurate dating is not possible or the cervix is "unripe", the patient should be managed conservatively with semiweekly clinical visits. The clinician should record the dilation of the cervix, fundal height, maternal weight, presence or absence of hypertension, and estimated fetal weight. Daily breast massage with warm compresses or nipple stimulation at or beyond term may promote the onset of spontaneous labor.

Fetal assessment tests should include fetal movement charting daily and fetal heart rate testing semiweekly. A reactive nonstress test (two or more adequate accelerations of the baseline fetal heart rate during a 20-40 min period) should be repeated within the next week. A nonreactive result should be repeated that same day, or a contraction stress test should be performed. The nonstress test provides useful information but remains a test of convenience. The contraction stress test is used at many institutions as the initial antepartum fetal heart rate test at 42 weeks and is recommended if undelivered by the 43rd week.

The observation of fetal activity and fetal heart rate patterns during the stress of spontaneous or oxytocin-induced uterine contractions provides useful information. The absence of fetal heart rate decelerations coincident with uterine activity is reassuring; but when decelerations are detected, they suggest fetal compromise from cord compression or uteroplacental insufficiency. Evidence for an active fetus requires the mother's perception of four or more vigorous fetal movements per hour beginning as early as the 40th completed week. Fetal inactivity (three or fewer movements per hour for two consecutive hours) requires further investigation.

A 20-minute period of visualization of intrauterine contents by real-time ultrasonography may also be useful, with specific consideration given to the presence of any fetal malformations (anencephaly), gross fetal body movements, fetal respiratory movements, and amniotic fluid volume. Amniotic fluid may be characterized as being adequate, pockets, or oligohydramnios (2 cm depth or less). Gross fetal body movement involves simultaneous trunk and lower limb motion, while fetal respiratory movements involve a rhythmic movement of the diaphragm.

Oligohydramnios is a warning sign of an increased risk of meconium, fetal acidosis, perinatal morbidity and mortality, and birth asphyxia. Traditionally associated with placental insufficiency, oligohydramnios may be difficult to determine by clinical examination because of a large fetus and the normally expected reduced quantity of amniotic fluid. Visualization using ultrasonography is quite helpful in predicting fetal postmaturity.

An amniocentesis to search for meconium or fetal lung testing is not recommended because of the decreased fluid and questionable value of test interpretation. Experience with amnioscopy to search for meconium is quite limited.

Intrapartum Management

If the cervix is ripe or there are any abnormal findings on clinical examination or fetal testing, delivery with optimal fetal monitoring is recommended. A trial of labor is appropriate if the fetus is presenting cephalically. We are now offering our patients the option of receiving a dose of prostaglandin E_2 gel on the cervical os when the cervix is unripe (Bishop score less than 5), assuming there is no contraindication to labor. The patient should be instructed that once labor begins, she should come to the hospital for electronic fetal heart rate monitoring. Once easily palpable, the amniotic membranes should be ruptured to permit internal monitoring of the fetal heart rate and uterine activity.

Most persons who desire a vaginal birth after a prior cesarean section decide on a repeat operation if undelivered by 42 weeks. There is an approximately 20% chance of a primary cesarean section or need for forceps delivery. This would be explained by the increased incidence of cephalopelvic disproportion and fetal distress. Any evidence of fetal distress requires observation and prompt delivery if a fetal heart rate abnormality is noted.

The physician caring for the baby should be notified in advance of the anticipated delivery. If meconium is present, a DeLee suction trap should be used to clear the upper airways immediately after delivery of the baby's head. After delivery of the remainder of the body, the upper airway including the vocal cords should be inspected and suctioned for the presence of any retained meconium.

Any infant with physical findings of postmaturity requires close observation, since those with birth asphyxia, hypoglycemia, and hypocalcemia often require admission to the intensive care nursery.

Suggested Readings

First Trimester Bleeding

Anderson SG: Management of threatened abortion with real-time sonography: Obstet. Gynecol. 55:259, 1980.

Barnes AB, Wennberg CCN, Barnes BA: Ectopic pregnancy: Incidence and review of determinant factors. Obstet. Gynecol. Surv. 38:345, 1983.

Gleicher N, Giglia RV, Deppe G, et al: Direct diagnosis of unruptured ectopic pregnancy by real-time ultrasonography. Obstet. Gynecol. 61:425, 1983.

Hertz JB: Diagnostic procedures in threatened abortion. Obstet. Gynecol. 64:223, 1984.

Hertz JB, Heisterberg L: The outcome of pregnancy after threatened abortion. Acta Obstet. Gynecol. Scand. 64:151, 1985.

Abnormal Pap Smear

Ostergard DR, Nieberg RK: Evaluation of abnormal cervical cytology during pregnancy with colposcopy. Am. J. Obstet. Gynecol. 134:756, 1979.

Ostergard DR: The effect of pregnancy on the cervical squamocolumnar junction in patients with abnormal cervical cytology. Am. J. Obstet. Gynecol. 134:759, 1979.

Leiman G, Harrison NA, Rubin A: Pregnancy following conization of the cervix: Complications related to cone size. Am. J. Obstet. Gynecol. 136:14, 1980.

Lee RB, Neglia W, Park RC: Cervical carcinoma in pregnancy. Obstet. Gynecol. 58:584, 1981.

Hacker NF, Berek JS, Lagasse LD, et al: Carcinoma of the cervix associated with pregnancy. Obstet. Gynecol. 59:735, 1982.

Nisker JA, Shubat M: Stage IB cervical carcinoma and pregnancy: Report of 49 cases. Am. J. Obstet. Gynecol. 145:203, 1983.

Rh Isoimmunization

Harman CR, Manning FA, Bowman JM, et al: Severe Rh disease - Poor outcome is not inevitable. Am. J. Obstet. Gynecol. 145:823, 1983.

Scott JR, Kochenour NK, Larkin RM, et al: Changes in the management of severely Rh-immunized patients. Am. J. Obstet. Gynecol. 149:336, 1984.

Quinlan RW, Buhi WC, Cruz AC: Fetal pulmonary maturity in isoimmunized pregnancies. Am. J. Obstet. Gynecol. 148:787, 1984.

Berkowitz RL, Chitkara U, Goldberg JD, et al: Intrauterine intravascular transfusions for severe red blood cell isoimmunization: Ultrasound-guided percutaneous approach. Am. J. Obstet. Gynecol. 155:574, 1986.

Management of isoimmunization in pregnancy. ACOG Tech. Bull. 90, January, 1986.

Caine ME, Mueller-Heubach E: Kell sensitizationin pregnancy. Am. J. Obstet. Gynecol. 154:85, 1986.

Sokol M, MacGregor S, Pielet B, et al: Percutaneous umbilical transfusion in severe rhesus isoimmunization: Resolution of fetal hydrops. Am. J. Obstet. Gynecol. 157:1369, 1987.

Premature Labor

Barden TP, Peter JB, Merkatz IR: Ritodrine hydrochloride: A betamimetic agent for use in preterm labor I. Pharmacology, clinical history, administration, side effects, and safety. Obstet. Gynecol. 56:1, 1980.

Creasy RK, Golbus MS, Laros RK, et al: Oral ritodrine maintenance in the treatment of preterm labor. Am. J. Obstet. Gynecol. 137:212, 1980.

Minkoff H: Prematurity: Infection as an etiologic factor. Obstet. Gynecol. 62:137, 1983.

Castle BM, Turnbull AC: The presence or absence of fetal breathing movements predicts the outcome of preterm labour. Lancet 2:471, 1983.

Finley J, Katz M, Rojas-Perez M, et al: Cardiovascular consequences of beta-agonist tocolysis: An echocardiographic study. Obstet. Gynecol. 64:787, 1984.

Caritis SN, Toig G, Heddinger LA, et al: A double-blind study comparing ritodrine and terbutaline in the treatment of preterm labor. Am. J. Obstet. Gynecol. 150:7, 1984.

Hatjis CG, Nelson LH, Meis PJ, et al: Addition of magnesium sulfate improves effectiveness of ritodrine in preventing premature delivery. Am. J. Obstet. Gynecol. 150:142, 1984.

Carr-Hill RA, Hall MH: The repetition of spontaneous preterm labour. Br. J. Obstet. Gynaecol. 92:921, 1985.

Gravett MG, Hummel D, Eschenbach DA, et al: Preterm labor associated with subclinical amniotic fluid infection and with bacterial vaginosis. Obstet. Gynecol. 67:229, 1986.

Gonik B, Creasy RK: Preterm labor: Its diagnosis and management. Am. J. Obstet. Gynecol. 154:3, 1986.

Katz M, Newman RB, Gill PJ: Assessment of uterine activity in ambulatory patients at high risk of preterm labor and delivery. Am. J. Obstet. Gynecol. 154:44, 1986.

Morrison JC, Martin JN, Martin RW, et al: Prevention of preterm birth by ambulatory assessment of uterine activity: A randomized study. Am. J. Obstet. Gynecol. 156:536, 1987.

Preterm Rupture of Membranes

Garite TJ, Freeman RK, Linzey EM, et al: Prospective randomized study of corticosteroids in the management of premature rupture of the membranes and the premature gestation. Am. J. Obstet. Gynecol. 141:508, 1981.

Gibbs DS, Blanco JD: Premature rupture of the membranes. Obstet. Gynecol. 60:671, 1982.

Curet LB, Rao V, Zachman RD, et al: Association between ruptured membranes, tocolytic therapy, and respiratory distress syndrome. Am. J. Obstet. Gynecol. 148:263, 1984.

Ismail MA, Zinaman MJ, Lowensohn RI, et al: The significance of C-reactive protein levels in women with premature rupture of membranes. Am. J. Obstet. Gynecol. 151:541, 1985.

Garite TJ: Premature rupture of the membranes: The enigma of the obstetrician. Am. J. Obstet. Gynecol. 151:1001, 1985.

Vintzileos AM, Feinstein SJ, Lodeiro JG, et al: Fetal biophysical profile and the effect of premature rupture of the membranes. Obstet. Gynecol. 67:818, 1986.

Monif GRG, Hume R, Goodlin RC: Neonatal considerations in the management of premature rupture of the fetal membranes. Obstet. Gynecol. Surv. 41:531, 1986.

Druzin ML, Toth M, Ledger WJ: Nonintervention in premature rupture of the amniotic membranes. Surg. Gynecol. Obstet. 163:5, 1986.

King JC, Mitzner W, Butterfield AB, et al: Effect of induced oligohydramnios on fetal lung development. Am. J. Obstet. Gynecol. 154:823, 1986.

Vintzileos AM, Bors-Koefoed R, Pelegano JF, et al: The use of fetal biophysical profile improves pregnancy outcome in premature rupture of the membranes. Am. J. Obstet. Gynecol. 157:236, 1987.

Garite TJ, Keegan KA, Freeman RK, et al: A randomized trial of ritodrine tocolysis versus expectant management in patients with premature rupture of membranes at 25 to 30 weeks of gestation. Am. J. Obstet. Gynecol. 157:388, 1987.

Bottoms SF, Welch RA, Zador IE, et al: Clinical interpretation of ultrasound measurements in preterm pregnancies with premature rupture of the membranes. Obstet. Gynecol. 69:358, 1987.

Corticosteroids to Enhance Fetal Lung Maturity

Liggins GC, Howie RN: A controlled trial of antepartum glucocorticoid treatment for prevention of the respiratory distress syndrome in premature infants. Pediatrics 51:515, 1972.

Collaborative group on antenatal steroid therapy: Effect of antenatal dexamethasone administration on the prevention of respiratory distress syndrome. Am. J. Obstet. Gynecol. 141:276, 1981.

Garite TJ, Freeman RK, Linzey EM, et al: Prospective randomized study of corticosteroids in the management of premature rupture of the membranes and the premature gestation. Am. J. Obstet. Gynecol. 141:508, 1981.

Farrell PM, Engle MJ, Zachman RD, et al: Amniotic fluid phospholipids after maternal administration of dexamethasone. Am. J. Obstet. Gynecol. 145:484, 1983.

Collaborative group on antenatal steroid therapy: Effects of antenatal dexamethaxone administration in the infant: Long-term follow-up. J. Pediatr. 104:259, 1984.

Ferguson JE, Hensleigh PA, Gill P: Effects of betamethasone on white blood cells in patients with premature rupture of the membranes and preterm labor. Obstet. Gynecol. 150:439, 1984.

Multifetal Gestation

Weekes ARL, Menzies DN, de Boer CH: The relative efficacy of bed rest, cervical suture, and no treatment in the management of twin pregnancy. Br. J. Obstet. Gynaecol. 84:161, 1977.

Ron-El R, Caspi E, Schreyer P, et al: Triplet and quadruplet pregnancies and management. Obstet. Gynecol. 57:458, 1981.

Chervenak FA, Johnson RE, Berkowitz RL, et al: Intrapartum external version of the second twin. Obstet Gynecol. 62:160, 1983.

Socol ML, Tamura RK, Sabbagha RE, et al: Diminished biparietal diameter and abdominal circumference growth in twins. Obstet. Gynecol. 64:235, 1984.

Rayburn W, Lavin J, Miodovnik M, et al: Multifetal gestation: Time interval between delivery of the first and second twin. Obstet. Gynecol. 63:502, 1984.

Saunders MC, Dick JS, Brown IM, et al: The effects of hospital admission for bed rest on the duration of twin pregnancy: A randomised trial. Lancet 2:793,1985.

Bell D, Johansson D, McLean FH, et al: Birth asphyxia, trauma, and mortality in twins: Has cesarean section improved outcome? Am. J. Obstet. Gynecol. 154:235, 1986.

Landy HJ, Weiner S, Corson SL, et al: The "vanishing twin": Ultrasonograhic assessment of fetal disappearance in the first trimester. Am. J. Obstet Gynecol. 155:14, 1986.

Lodeiro JG, Vintzileos AM, Feinstein SJ, et al: Fetal biophysical profile in twin gestations. Obstet. Gynecol. 67:824, 1986.

Rattan PK, Knuppel RA, O'Brien WF, et al: Cesarean delivery of the second twin after vaginal delivery of the first twin. Am. J. Obstet. Gynecol. 154:936, 1986.

Third Trimester Bleeding

Newton ER, Barss V, Cetrulo CL: The epidemiology and clinical history of asymptomatic midtrimester placenta previa. Am. J. Obstet. Gynecol. 148:743, 1984.

Silver R, Depp R, Sabbagha RE, et al: Placenta previa: Aggresive expectant management. Am. J. Obstet. Gynecol. 150:15, 1984.

D'Angelo LJ, Irwin LF: Conservative management of placenta previa: A cost-benefit analysis. Am. J. Obstet. Gynecol. 149:320, 1984.

Chervenak FA, Lee Y, Hendler MA, et al: Role of attempted vaginal delivery in the management of placenta previa. Obstet. Gynecol. 64:798, 1984.

Abdella TN, Sibai BM, Hays JM, et al: Relationship of hypertensive disease to abruptio placentae. Obstet. Gynecol. 3:365, 1984.

Hertz JB: Diagnostic procedures in threatened abortion. Obstet. Gynecol. 64:223, 1984.

Clark SL, Koonings PP, Phelan JP: Placenta previa/accreta and prior cesarean section. Obstet. Gynecol. 66:89, 1985.

McShane PM, Heyl PS, Epstein MF: Maternal and perinatal morbidity resulting from placenta previa. Obstet. Gynecol. 65:176, 1985.

Karegard M, Gennser G: Incidence and recurrence rate of abruptio placentae in Sweden. Obstet. Gynecol. 67:523, 1986.

Sholl JS: Abruptio placentae: Clinical mangement in nonacute cases. Am. J. Obstet. Gynecol. 156:40, 1987.

Nyberg DA, Cyr DR, Mack LA, et al: Sonographic spectrum of placental abruption. Am. J. Radiol. 148:161, 1987.

Sholl JS: Abruptio placentae: Clinical management in nonacute cases. Am. J. Obstet. Gynecol. 156:40, 1987.

Postdates

Green JN, Paul RH: The value of amniocentesis in prolonged pregnancy. Obstet. Gynecol. 51:293, 1978.

Freeman RK, Garite TJ, Modanlou H, et al: Postdate pregnancy: Utilization of contraction stress testing for primary fetal surveillance. Am. J. Obstet. Gynecol. 140:128, 1981.

Rayburn WF, Motley ME, Stempel LE, et al: Antepartum prediction of the postmature infant. Obstet. Gynecol. 60:148, 1982.

Eden RD, Gergely RZ, Schifrin BS, et al: Comparison of antepartum testing schemes for the management of the postdate pregnancy. Am. J. Obstet. Gynecol. 144:683, 1982.

Leveno KJ,Quirk JG, Cunningham FG, et al: Prolonged pregnancy I. Observations concerning the causes of fetal distress. Am. J. Obstet. Gynecol. 150:465, 1984.

Phelan JP, Platt LD, Yeh SY, et al: The role of ultrasound assessment of amniotic fluid volume in the management of the postdate pregnancy. Am. J. Obstet. Gynecol. 151:304, 1985.

Lagrew DC, Freeman RK: Management of postdate pregnancy. Am. J. Obstet. Gynecol. 154:8, 1986.

Johnson JM, Harman CR, Lange IR, et al: Biophysical profile scoring in the management of the postterm pregnancy: An analysis of 307 patients. Am. J. Obstet. Gynecol. 154:269, 1986.

Shime J, Librach CL, Gare DJ, et al: The influence of prolonged pregnancy on infant development at one and two years of age: A prospective controlled study. Am. J. Obstet. Gynecol. 154:341, 1986.

Dyson DC, Miller PD, Armstrong MA: Management of prolonged pregnancy: Induction of labor versus antepartum fetal testing. Am. J. Obstet. Gynecol. 156:928, 1987.

Bochner CJ, Medearis AL, Ross MG, et al: The role of antepartum testing in the management of postterm pregnancies with heavy meconium in early labor. Obstet. Gynecol. 69:903, 1987.

Chapter 4

Perinatal Infections

Common Vaginal Infections

A vaginal discharge is commonly encountered during pregnancy from hormonal effects and does not necessarily signify ruptured membranes or an inflammatory process. Most cases of infectious vaginitis result from Candida albicans, Trichomonas vaginalis, or Gardnerella vaginalis. Cervicitis, caused primarily by Neisseria gonorrhoeae, Chlamydia trachomatis, and Herpes simplex, is responsible for most patients' complaints of vaginal discharge. A thorough assessment and an accurate diagnosis are important steps in effecting a cure, since an inaccurate or non-specific diagnosis can lead to the majority of treatment failures.

Candida

Candida infections are at least ten times more frequent in pregnant than nonpregnant women. The increased estrogen production during pregnancy and increased glycogen content of the vagina favor growth. Infection may be asymptomatic, but most often produces a whitish discharge associated with pruritus and burning of the vulva. Microscopic examination of any vaginal discharge is imperative, with the wet mount having a sensitivity of 40-80%. Sensitivity is improved by adding a drop of 10% potassium hydroxide (KOH) to the wet mount, which dissolves epithelial cells and other debris and allows earlier visualization of the diagnostic blastospores.

Miconazole nitrate cream or vaginal suppositories daily for one week will usually alleviate the symptoms, but recurrence is common. It is worthwhile for a patient who has had one documented infection during pregnancy to be offered one weekly application of miconazole cream for the duration of the gestation to prevent symptomatic recurrence. A five day course of oral nystatin tablets, 4 times daily, may be helpful in preventing recurrence, because Candida reside in the lower intestinal tract and are a source of infection of the perineum and vagina. There are no known adverse effects from either of these drugs used during pregnancy. Rare candidal infections of the placenta are associated with high prematurity and perinatal death rates. Neonatal oral candidiasis and dermatitis are common lesions where there has been contact with the mother at delivery. The oral lesions are recognized as neonatal thrush and usually resolve without incident when treated with antifungal agents.

Trichomonas

Trichomoniasis is one of the most frequently occurring sexually-acquired diseases, and it is often not diagnosed until there is a profuse, foul smelling vaginal discharge or an abnormal pap smear. However, up to half of infected women may be asymptomatic. The diagnosis is confirmed by identifying motile, flagellated organisms using 45 x magnification. The current treatment is metronidazole, 250 mg tablets three times daily for seven days. A single 2 gm dose is thought to have a cure rate of 97%, assuming there is no further reinfection. This dosing regimen would improve the compliance rate while lowering costs. Concurrent single dose therapy of the male sexual partners is recommended. If this 2 gm dose fails, 500 mg twice daily for one week should be effective. Resistance to the metronidazole is rare. The gastrointestinal side effects are usually well tolerated.

Metronidazole has not been shown to be teratogenic in either human or animal studies, but the manufacturer recommends that use of this drug be limited to the second and third trimesters. The understandable concern about the theoretic risk to the fetus can be countered by a strong argument for metronidazole therapy in pregnancy based on the role trichomoniasis and its associated anaerobic bacterial overgrowth may play in premature rupture of the membranes and postpartum endometritis.

Bacterial Vaginosis

Bacterial vaginosis is the newer terminology for the disease formerly designated as "nonspecific vaginitis". Both Gardnerella (Hemophilus) vaginalis and anaerobic bacterial overgrowth characterize the entity bacteriologically. A symbiotic relation between G. vaginalis and anaerobic bacterial overgrowth in the vagina is responsible for the signs and symptoms which consist primarily of an increase in vaginal secretions and "fishy" odor. The diagnosis is confirmed microscopically on saline wet prep by identifying "clue cells" (vaginal epithelial cells with indistinctive cell borders obscured by a large number of attached organisms) and by noting the strong amine odor after alkalinization of the secretions with 10% potassium hydroxide.

Although controversy remains, most authorities feel that the male sexual partner does not need to be treated. Metronidazole in a dose of 500 mg twice daily for seven days has proven to be highly effective; however, single dose therapy using 2 gm is thought to be less effective. Oral ampicillin therapy has also provided good cure rates.

Group B Streptococci

Group B streptococci are common bacteria colonizing the vagina in approximately 15% of pregnant women. The actual attack rate is quite low, however. Group B streptococci are a leading cause of neonatal sepsis with an attack rate ranging between 0.35 and 5.4 per 1,000 live births and a mortality rate exceeding 5%. Early diagnosis and treatment are fundamental to improve the outcome of a septic neonate.

Antenatal screening of all pregnant women for Group B streptococci colonization has not been routine on the basis of a very low ratio of neonatal sepsis to colonized mothers (about 0.7%). Studies have demonstrated that the intermittently treated mother often reverts to a carrier state shortly after the antibiotic was discontinued.

Screening for Group B streptococci colonization and treatment with penicillin if culture-positive has been reserved for those cases when premature labor, preterm ruptured membranes, ruptured membranes for more than 24 hours, intrapartum fever, or prior affected newborn infant has been diagnosed. It is extremely difficult to determine which neonates are infected because obvious clinical signs, such as pneumonia, are usually not apparent at birth.

Chlamydia

Chlamydia trachomatis is the most common cause of sexually transmitted disease. It is a frequent cause of maternal bartholinitis, endocervicitis, and acute urethritis, as well as neonatal conjunctivitis and pneumonia. Routine monoclonal antibody testing or culturing at the initial prenatal visit does not appear to be cost effective. Select screening is considered to be worthwhile if there is recurrent abortion, premature labor, preterm ruptured membranes, sexually transmitted infection, abnormal pap smear, or a prior poor obstetrical history. Concurrent infection with C. Trachomatis should be suspected when gonorrhea of the genital tract is diagnosed. Penicillin and its derivatives are effective treatment for gonorrhea, whereas Chlamydia responds to erythromycin or tetracycline. When a chlamydial infection is recognized in a patient, her sexual partner should also be treated with erythromycin or tetracycline.

In utero transmission is not known to occur, but an infant delivered vaginally has a 60-70% risk of acquiring the infection. Approximately 25-50% of exposed infants will develop conjunctivitis in the first two weeks and 10-20% will develop pneumonia in the first 3-4 months. Although controversial, most of the current literature suggests there is no increase in adverse pregnancy outcomes when chlamydial infection is not treated during pregnancy. However, treatment of chlamydial cervicitis with erythromycin during the late weeks of pregnancy is an effective means of preventing neonatal conjunctivitis and pneumonia. Erythromycin ointment applied routinely to the infant's eyes at delivery is effective prophylactic treatment of chlamydial and gonococcal ophthalmia.

Urinary Tract Infection

Asymptomatic bacteriuria is reported to occur in 2-12% of all pregnancies. It is most common in black, multiparous patients with sickle cell trait but may also be found in women with diabetes, obesity, history of UTI, urinary tract anomalies, renal stones, and urethral catheterization. Approximately one-fourth of women with asymptomatic bacteriuria will subsequently develop a symptomatic urinary tract infection. Bacteriuria may be a manifestation of an underlying chronic renal disease and is associated with a higher incidence of perinatal loss and low birth weight infants. Any increased risk of premature labor may relate to the release of prostaglandins from the bacterial walls.

Diagnosis

Each patient should have a urine culture or urinalysis taken during the initial prenatal visit. A clean midstream urine specimen containing more than 100,000 colonies of the same pathogen per milliliter of urine is diagnostic of bacteriuria. Contamination of the specimen during collection should be suspected with a smaller colony count or multiple organisms. After an initial negative culture, less than 1.5% of those patients will subsequently acquire a urinary infection before delivery.

Therapy

Ampicillin, sulfonamides, nitrofurantoin, and cephalosporins have been used successfully to treat urinary tract infections. A 10 day course of ampicillin (500 mg 4 times daily) or macrodantin (50 mg 4 times daily) is recommended. Macrodantin should be avoided if there is evidence of a hemolytic anemia in women whose erythrocytes are deficient in G6PD (2% of black women are homozygous for this x-linked enzyme deficiency) and substituted with ampicillin beyond 36 weeks, because of hyperbilirubinemia which may occur in newborn infants with in utero exosure to sulfa drugs.

Symptoms usually subside within 2 days after beginning therapy, but the medication should be continued for at least 7 days. A urine culture is recommended within 1 week following completion of the drug therapy. If the culture remains positive, the proper drug should be chosen according to the sensitivity pattern of the isolated organism.

Hospitalization for a urinary tract infection is necessary when there are systemic manifestations of upper urinary tract problems. Along with the intravenous administration of ampicillin, the patient should be watched carefully for any signs of septic shock. A transient decrease in glomerular filtration and a transient form of hemolytic anemia may appear. Acute respiratory distress may develop rarely and is felt to be mediated by bacterial endotoxins. If the patient does not show a response to ampicillin within 24 hrs, an aminoglycoside should be added. Alternatively, if sensitivities are available, they may be utilized to choose a more appropriate antibiotic. Either chronic low dose antibiotic suppression (Macrodantin 50 mg twice daily or 100 mg HS) or repeat cultures on a monthly basis are necessary in any pregnant patient with pyelonephritis.

If the culture becomes positive, chronic suppression should be undertaken. Screening for sickle cell disease is necessary for black gravidas who develop pyelonephritis. Any patient with persistent, recurrent, or very severe urinary tract infections during pregnancy should be evaluated in the postpartum period. An intravenous pyelogram, creatinine clearance determination, and urine culture should be obtained.

Herpes Simplex

The relative infrequency of neonatal herpes (2 in 7,500 live births) has made it difficult to study the disease thoroughly. It has been reported that the infection rate of infants born to mothers with symptomatic genital Herpes simplex is 50%, with manifestations ranging from subclinical to cutaneous to disseminatal (visceral) disease, with or without CNS involvement. Of those infected systemically, 60% will die and of those who survive, many are impaired neurologically. The mean onset of symptoms in newborn infants is 6 days, although those who are systemically infected may have delayed onset of clinical signs. The first signs of neonatal herpes infection are variable and range from lethargy to seizures or overwhelming systemic disease.

Antepartum Screening

Virus isolation on tissue culture remains the standard diagnostic procedure. Cultures of the cervix, posterior vaginal fornix, and vulva should be obtained if there is a history of genital herpes, sexual contact during pregnancy with a person having any visibly suspicious genital lesion, or any suspicious vulvar lesion. Cervical cultures should be performed weekly beginning at the 36th week. Cultures are positive in 92% of colonized cases after 4 days incubation.

If cultures have not been done previously and patient is suspected by history or physical examination to have genital herpes, a pap smear may be helpful and provide information relatively quickly. Cervico-vaginal smears have been reported to detect 75% of specimens positive for Herpes simplex on culture. Negative cytologic findings do not rule out herpes, however.

Most genital herpes during pregnancy is a recurrence of prior disease. External genital lesions are usually preceded by prodromal symptoms such as pruritus, numbness, pain, burning, or paresthesias. The typical course of genital herpes infection involves a prodrome of 1-2 days, vesicle/pustule stage of 2 days, wet ulcer stage of 3 days, and dry crust stage of 7 days. Virus shedding occurs during the 5-day vesicle/pustule/wet ulcer period, and the mean interval betweeen recurrences is 59 days but may be less than 21 days.

Recently, recognition of the low rate of asymptomatic viral shedding (1.4% at term), the short duration of viral shedding during an attack, and the less than 5% incidence of neonatal infection among infants born to mothers with asymptomatic viral shedding has led some investigators to advocate the abandonment of weekly cultures. These authorities recommend that cesarean section be reserved for individuals with symptomatic infection at the time of or during the few days preceding labor and that vaginal delivery be allowed for all others. While the data presented by this group appears to be very promising, weekly cultures continue to be performed on the authors' services pending confirmation of the safety of eliminating this practice by other investigators.

Local Therapy

Treatment goals include relief of symptoms and promoting re-epithelialization. This involves frequent washing with soap and water, thorough drying (blow dryer or heat lamp may be useful), and dusting with baby powder or corn starch. Any benefit or risk from topical acyclovir to nonmucocutaneous areas during pregnancy is presently unknown.

Mode of Delivery

Cesarean Section
Cesarean section is recommended if 1) the mother has active genital herpetic lesions at the time of delivery and membranes are intact or ruptured less than 6 hrs, or 2) the mother has had a recent positive culture or pap smear for herpes. Individual discretion is necessary if there are grossly obvious lesions in the lower genital tract and the membranes have been ruptured for more than 6 hrs.

Vaginal Delivery
Vaginal delivery is recommended if 1) the lesions are seen and membranes are ruptured more than 4-6 hrs before the anticipated time of delivery, or 2) the two weekly cultures immediately preceding delivery were negative and the mother has no genital herpes at term. If genital herpes is suspected, fetal scalp electrode placement or scalp pH determinations should not be performed until an active infection is ruled out.

Alternatively
If weekly cultures are not performed, any gravida with symptoms of recurrent infection or visible lesions should be delivered by cesarean section. The remaining patients should have a culture taken at the time of labor to detect asymptomatic infection and should be delivered vaginally.

Postpartum Infection Control Measures

Mother with Proven or Clinically Suspected Genital Herpes at Term
The Center for Disease Control Guidelines do not require isolation of these mothers on the antepartum and postpartum floors. However, from a practical point of view, other patients generally become upset when placed in a room with a woman with an active herpes infection. Therefore, isolation is usually practiced at the authors' institutions,

using wound and skin precautions. Perineal pads, genital dressings, and bed linen should be double-bagged. The mother may handle and feed her infant if she is out of bed (to reduce a chance of contact with potentially contaminated bed linen), gowned, and follows thorough handwashing techniques. The infant should be isolated with wound and skin precautions. Contaminated articles should be double-bagged.

The newborn infant may be brought to the mother under supervised conditions as above. Rooming-in is acceptable after the mother has been taught appropriate protective measures. Circumcision should be delayed in proven and suspected cases. A joint committee from the American College of Obstetricians and Gynecologists and the American Academy of Pediatrics recommends that these babies be cultured for the virus (urine, conjunctiva, nasopharynx, other suspicious sites) and have liver function tests and spinal fluid examinations.

Mothers with Non-Oral, Non-Genital Lesions at Delivery

Cover maternal lesions at all times. Wound and skin precautions with isolation are necessary for the mother. The infant does not require isolation initially but should be isolated and placed on wound and skin precautions after contact with the mother. If there are no lesions in the area of the breasts, the mother may breast feed; otherwise, she may pump to establish and maintain milk flow. This milk should be discarded until the breast lesions are healed.

Mothers with Oral Lesions Only

Exposure to oral herpes (type 1) may be as devastating as genital herpes (type 2) to the neonate. She should cover her lesions with a mask or gauze until they are crusted and should refrain from kissing and nuzzling her infant. The infant does not require isolation, however.

Mothers with Two Negative Cervical Cultures Preceding Delivery and No Evidence of Infection at Delivery

There is no need to isolate the mother or baby or limit their interaction. Infants who are suspected of exposure, but who are handled according to the preceding guidelines and who display no signs or symptoms of disease may be discharged with the mother. The primary source of follow-up care must be notified. Maternal education must take place to allow prompt recognition of signs of infection in the infant and early institution of therapy.

For Medical or Nursing Personnel with Oral Lesions Only

Oral lesions should be covered with a mask and/or gauze until they are crusted. Any infant contact with a lesion should be avoided. Careful handwashing is essential to avoid secondary contamination after an individual has touched an infected area.

For Medical or Nursing Personnel with Hand Lesions

Contact with infants is prohibited until lesions clear.

Viral Hepatitis

Hepatitis B is the most common cause of viral hepatitis in pregnancy. Maternal mortality is low in well-nourished populations and is the same as for nonpregnant populations. Mortality rates are alarmingly high in poorly nourished persons. The incidence of abortion and premature labor are increased with Hepatitis B, and neonatal infection may occur transplacentally or by direct contact with the mother during and after delivery. Recent epidemiologic studies suggest that it is difficult to distinguish individuals at high risk for asymptomatic infection on the basis of clinical criteria. Therefore, in certain high risk populations, universal screening may be appropriate.

Other cases of liver dysfunction include noninfectious hepatitis (drug-related), CMV and other virus infections, gallstones, as well as the following:

First Trimester:
   hyperemesis gravidarum, drug reactions
Second Trimester:
   cirrhosis, pyelonephritis, exacerbation of chronic liver disease
Third Trimester:
   cholestasis of pregnancy, eclampsia, preeclampsia, cirrhosis, fatty liver of pregnancy, pyelonephritis

Characteristics of Hepatitis A, B, and non-A, non-B are compared in Table 4.1. The laboratory diagnosis of these liver disorders presenting during the third trimester are shown in Table 4.2.

Forms of Viral Hepatitis

Hepatitis B is the most common form during pregnancy. Mothers who have Hepatitis B surface antigen (HB Ag) without antibody have had a prior infection or immunization and are currently immune, while those who have detectable surface antigen (HB Ag) without antibody have active infection or are chronic carriers. Mothers who are also carriers of e antigens and who lack the e antibody are infectious and may transmit the virus to the fetus.

Infants born to mothers who are chronic carriers of Hepatitis B Ag may have severe or lethal hepatitis during the first 4 months of infancy, and these infants commonly become chronic carriers. While infection rates are higher for infants whose mothers become infected in the third trimester, these infants usually experience milder disease. Hepatitis B immune globulin (HBIG) and Hepatitis B vaccine should be administered to decrease the incidence of maternal disease.

Transplacental Hepatitis A infection has not been reported. However, neonatal infection does occur. Therefore, infants born to mothers with active Hepatitis A infection should be treated with Immune Specific Globulin. There is little information about perinatal transmission of non-A non-B hepatitis.

Table 4.1
Forms of Viral Hepatitis*

Characteristics	Hepatitis A	Hepatitis B	Non-A, Non-B
Prior terminology	Infectious hepatitis	Serum hepatitis	Unrecognized
Virus type	RNA	DNA	appears to be similar to B
Incubation time	15-50 days	30-180 days	30-160 days
Transmission route	Fecal-oral	Parenteral or body fluids	Parenteral, close contacts
Diagnosis	HA antibody IgM and IgG types	HB_SAg, HB_CAg HB_SAb, HB_eAg	By exclusion, most commonly seen post-transfusion
Maximum infectivity	Prodrome	Prodrome or HB_SAg carriers	Probably prodrome
Acute clinical forms	Asymptomatic to fulminant	Asymptomatic to fulminant	Asymptomatic to fulminant
Incidence of chronicity	0%	5-10%	More than 10%
Chronic clinical forms	None	Chronic persistent hepatitis Chronic active hepatitis Asymptomatic carrier	Chronic persistent Chronic active Asymptomatic carrier
Transmission risk to infant	Rare	1st & 2nd trimester: 10% 3rd trimester: 65%	Uncertain (little information)
Infant disease	Rare clinical hepatitis, (at 14-30 days of age) No carriers	Usually mild hepatitis rarely severe (at 20-120 days of age) Commonly become carriers	

Table 4.1 (Continued)

Characteristics	Hepatitis A	Hepatitis B
Prophylaxis for infant	ISG - only for infant of mother with acute infection	ISG - not useful
	HBIG - not useful	HBIG - useful at birth and at 3 mos.
		Vaccine - useful after HBIG(?)

*From Fallen, et al., pp 289-291.

Proposed Management

1. Institute appropriate isolation and precautions until type of hepatitis confirmed
2. Establish type by immunologic test
3. Determine need for contact prophylaxis with serum globulin preparations
4. Activity - determined by tolerance; rest encouraged
5. Diet - patient preference; parenteral if necessary, high protein
6. Antiemetics - phenothiazines may be used
7. Corticosteroids - not indicated
8. Notify pediatrician before anticipated delivery
9. Watch for any mental or sleep disturbance - impending coma
10. Treat any additional medical problems
11. Discharge from hospital after improvement in liver function tests
12. Attempts should be made at delivery to avoid aspiration by the infant of any maternal blood. Observe blood precautions for pre- and post delivery care if HB_SAg-positive
13. If the mother remains infected during delivery, breast feeding should be avoided. Handle blood- or lochia-soaked dressings with gloved hands and disinfect sitz baths
14. Among health care personnel, obstetricians and gynecologists are considered to be at average risk of acquiring Hepatitis B virus infection. Other hospital staff such as nurses, phlebotomists, and IV team personnel are at higher risk and are considered to be candidates for hepatitis vaccine, immunization which is effective and safe. No long-term side effects have been demonstrated from the use of this dead vaccine, and the duration of immunity is at least 3 yr in most recipients.

Table 4.2
Laboratory Diagnosis of Liver Disease in Third Trimester*

Condition	SGOT (IU/L)	Bilirubin (mg/100 ml)	Alkaline phosphatase
Normal pregnancy	Normal (2-35)	Normal (1.2) to slight increase	2 x increase (nl:30-96 IU/L)
Infectious hepatitis	500-1,000	1.5-5	2-3 x increase
Cholestasis of pregnancy	Normal	1.5-5	10 x increase
Toxemia	100-1,000	Sl increase	2-3 x increase
Gallstones	Normal to sl increase	Variable	3-10 x increase
Active cirrhoses and chronic active hepatitis	50-150	1.5-5	3 x increase
Fatty liver of pregnancy	300-500	1.5-10	3 x increase

*A liver biopsy can be performed during a cesarean section using a True-cut biopsy needle. There is no increased hepatic blood flow during pregnancy, so the risk of hemorrhage is the same. We recommend that the liver and gall bladder be palpated at the time of intra-abdominal surgery.

Acquired Immunodeficiency Syndrome

Acquired immunodeficiency syndrome (AIDS) is an infectious disease caused by a retrovirus known as human T-cell lymphotropic virus (HIV). The virus can be transmitted through sexual intercourse, contaminated needles, blood or blood product transfusion, or perinatally from mother to infant. A large increase in the prevalence of AIDS is expected over the next several years.

Perinatal Transmission
Several hundred cases of pediatric acquired immunodeficiency syndrome have been documented with a large percent resulting from perinatal transmission. Transmission of the virus may occur before, during, or after birth. The rate of perinatal transmission of the virus is unknown but may be up to 65% of exposed infants. The virus has been isolated from breast milk of infected women, and breast

feeding may be implicated as a mode of transmission. Most mothers are asymptomatic during pregnancy. Preliminary data suggest that there is an increase of spontaneous abortion, low birth weight, premature rupture of membranes, and premature delivery.

Dysmorphic syndrome with intrauterine HIV infection has been described recently in 20 infants and children with positive serologic tests. Growth failure, microcephaly, and craniofacial abnormalities have been found in those with positive serologic tests.

Follow-up examinations of infants at risk of developing AIDS are limited, but a slow rate of weight gain has been evident. The affected child's age at onset of symptoms does not necessarily correlate with the birth weight, mode of delivery, or status of membranes at the onset of labor.

Screening

The Center for Disease Control (CDC) has developed recommendations designed to reduce the risk of perinatal transmission. They recommend that women be counseled with regard to antibody testing if they are pregnant (or may become pregnant) and belong to any of the following groups:

1. IV drug abusers
2. those born in countries where heterosexual transmission is thought to play a major role
3. prostitutes
4. those who have been sex partners of IV drug abusers, bisexual men, men with hemophilia, men born in countries where heterosexual transmission is thought to play a major role, or men who otherwise have evidence of infection with HIV.

Counseling and testing of women who are not included in the above mentioned groups are not presently recommended by the CDC. If a woman requests screening, this service should be provided in accordance with the above recommendations. Counseling and testing must be conducted in a confidential environment. Testing for antibody should be performed with the woman's consent after counseling has been provided regarding risk of infection, interpretation of the test results, risk of transmission, and definite increased likelihood of disease among women infected with HIV. The screening antibody test for HIV is relatively inexpensive. If positive, confirmation should be obtained by the more expensive Western Blot test.

Counseling Infected Women

Women with positive results for HIV antibodies should be counseled regarding their own risk of AIDS and the risk of perinatal and sexual transmission.

1. Advise infected women to delay pregnancy until more is known regarding perinatal transmission.
2. Discourage drug use and advise against sharing needles.
3. Refer sex partners for counseling and testing.
4. Inform couples of protected sexual practices to reduce the risk of HIV transmission to uninfected partners. Encourage consistent and proper use of condoms.

5. Advise against breastfeeding.
6. Inform couple not to donate blood, organs, or sperm.

Infection Control

The precautions described below represent present practices which apply to preventing transmission of HIV and other bloodborne agents between infected patients and personnel who perform or assist in invasive procedures.

1. Wear gloves when touching mucous membranes or nonintact skin of all patients.
2. Utilize blood/body fluid precautions for all sero-positive patients during labor, delivery, and postpartum (e.g. gloves).
3. Use appropriate barrier precautions (e.g. gloves and gown) when handling the placenta or the infant until blood and amniotic fluid have been removed from infant's skin.
4. Use extraordinary care to prevent injuries caused by needles or sharp instruments during procedures.
5. Place linens in meltaway isolation bags, then special isolation linen bags before sending to laundry.
6. Wash hands properly and clean all equipment promptly with Chlorox solution (1:10 dilution).
7. Notify appropriate medical, nursing and other involved health care providers, and environmental services.

Genital Warts

Genital warts are caused by the human papillomavirus (HPV). They account for a large number of abnormal pap smears and relate to the later development of certain genital neoplasms. These viral infections are sexually transmitted. The latent period from exposure to development of flat, subclinical, epithelial proliferations averages about three months but can be much longer. The lesions appear around the vulva, introitus, perineum, anus, urethra, and cervix. Symptoms include itching, burning, pain, and tenderness, but cervical or vaginal HPV infections are usually asymptomatic. The external warts commonly recur, perhaps because of reinfection from sexual partners.

Management of these infections during pregnancy is difficult. The papillary lesions may proliferate on the vulva and vagina. Transmission to the infant may result from transplacental transmission of maternal infection, direct contact with the infected genital tract at delivery, or postnatal contact with an infected individual.

No specific antiviral therpy is widely available. Results with podophyllin have generally been poor with cure rates around 20%. Podophyllin, 5-fluorouracil, and immunotherapy should be avoided during pregnancy because of their systemic absorption and unknown effects on the developing fetus. Trichloracetic acid applied sparingly results in a higher cure rate, but repeated treatments may be necessary. Interferon has reportedly been effective in a controlled clinical trial, although it is not yet available for treatment of genital warts.

Recombinant DNA techniques may make this treatment more readily available.

Cryotherapy and electrocautery have reported cure rates of 63% and 90% respectively when performed in an outpatient setting with or without local anesthesia. Only visible lesions are amenable to treatment, however. Carbon dioxide laser therapy may be more effective, although controlled clinical trials are necessary. The time, cost, and morbidity rates from laser vaporization exceed those of other treatments, and advanced training in colposcopy and laser therapy is necessary.

Large and friable lesions may cause extensive vaginal damage and bleeding at delivery and necessitate cesarean section. There is currently no concensus regarding the protective benefit to the neonate of cesarean versus vaginal delivery. Because years of latency may precede the appearance of lesions, the risk for perinatally exposed children has been difficult to assess.

Gonorrhea

The incidence of gonococcal (GC) infections in pregnant patients has been reported to range from 3-6%. Most studies have involved indigent patient populations, and the incidence in the general population is probably lower. Acute salpingitis is a rare event after the third gestational month, because the cervical mucus plug blocks access of the ascending gram-negative diplococcus to the upper genital tract. However, the incidence of disseminated gonorrhea is higher during pregnancy.

Every pregnant woman should be cultured for gonorrhea at her initial prenatal visit, and again if recurrent infections remain a possibility. Prompt treatment is necessary to prevent maternal complications, infection of the patient's sexual partner, gonococcal ophthalmia neonatorium, and infection of the upper genital tract at the time of delivery. If the incidence of gonococcal infection in the third trimester is greater than 1% in the given population, the Center for Disease Control recommends routine repeat culturing at 34-36 weeks gestation.

Evaluation of a Positive Culture

Treatment for undisseminated, uncomplicated gonorrhea is the same as for the nonpregnant patient and may be undertaken on an outpatient basis, in accordance with the following guidelines:

1. Treat with adequate dose of an appropriate antibiotic as outlined in Table 4.3.
2. Reculture cervix and rectum as test of cure in 2 weeks and retreat if necessary. Culture again at 34-36 weeks gestation.
3. Examine and treat sexual contact(s).
4. Examine patient for other STD (chlamydia, syphilis, herpes) and treat accordingly.

5. Before delivery, notify pediatrician of maternal culture results. Consider GC cultures, serologic tests for syphilis, etc. on infant when appropriate.

Table 4.3
Single Dose Therapy for Women with Uncomplicated Gonorrhea (no signs or symptoms of bacteremia, endocarditis, arthritis, meningitis, ophthalmia)

Drugs of choice:
>Amoxicillin[a] 3 g po **plus** probenecid 1 g po
>OR
>Ceftriaxone[b,c] 125-250 mg IM (deltoid)

Alternatives:
>Penicillin G procaine 4.8 million U IM (divided into 2 injections at one visit) **plus** probenecid 1 g po
>Spectinomycin[b,d] 2 g IM
>Cefoxitin 2 g IM **plus** probenecid 1 g po

---

[a] Less effective against anal or pharyngeal gonorrhea
[b] Effective against penicillin-resistant strains; recommended in treatment failure
[c] Drug of choice for pharyngeal isolates
[d] Recommended for penicillin-allergic patients

Syphilis

Approximately 100,000 cases of adult syphilis and 300-400 cases of congenital syphilis are reported in the United States each year. Until recently, it has been felt that the spirochete did not cross the placenta until approximately 18 weeks gestation. It is now understood that the risk to the unborn child is present throughout gestation although the fetus is unable to mount an immune response to the spirochete until mid-gestation. This risk to the fetus is reduced when mothers have latent disease and decreased further with late syphilis. To minimize congenital disease, most states now require routine maternal screening for syphilis.

Diagnosis
Nonspecific antibody tests such as the VDRL or RPR are used for initial screening. When a positive serologic test is obtained, further evaluation as shown on the next page is indicated. A primary lesion consists of a chancre, usually on the labia. Secondary syphilis is characterized by a rash on the palmar and plantar surfaces, lymph-adenopathy, and other signs of systemic infection. Except for muco-

Evaluation of a Positive Serologic Test for Syphilis during Pregnancy

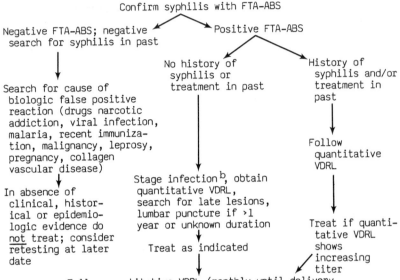

History, physical examination[b], careful review
of previous medical and obstetric records

Confirm syphilis with FTA-ABS

Negative FTA-ABS; negative ← → Positive FTA-ABS
search for syphilis in past

No history of   History of
syphilis or   syphilis and/or
treatment in past   treatment in
               past

Search for cause of
biologic false positive
reaction (drugs narcotic
addiction, viral infection,
malaria, recent immuniza-
tion, malignancy, leprosy,   Follow
pregnancy, collagen   quantitative
vascular disease)   VDRL

                Stage infection[b], obtain
In absence of   quantitative VDRL,
clinical, histor-   search for late lesions,
ical or epidemio-   lumbar puncture if >1
logic evidence do   year or unknown duration   Treat if quanti-
not treat; consider   tative VDRL
retesting at later   Treat as indicated   shows
date   increasing
                                             titer

Follow quantitative VDRL (monthly until delivery
then every 3 months for first year) 4-fold drop
in titer or return to nonreactive is regarded as
successful treatment

Examine neonate for clinical and serologic[c] evidence
(VDRL, FTA-ABS) of congenital syphilis at birth and
first weeks of life (maculopapular eruption, IUGR,
saddle nose, hepatosplenomegaly, jaundice)

---

[a]Serologic tests (RPR, VDRL) become positive 1-3 weeks after
infection. VDRL titer decreases until fixed low titer or
undetectable with sufficient therapy. FTA-ABS is less reliable as
an indicator of treatment efficacy and may remain positive for life.
[b]Darkfield exam of chancres or mucocutaneous lesions, or biopsy of
gumma may be helpful in staging.
[c]Positive serologic tests in neonates without stigmata of syphilis
may be either due to passive transfer of maternal antibodies or
prenatal infection. If adequate treatment of mother cannot be
documented, prompt treatment of seropositive infants is indicated
rather than waiting 3-6 months to see if antibody titer falls.
Variable sensitivity and specificity shown with FTA-ABS (IgM).

cutaneous lesions, late or latent infection is difficult to suspect on physical examination alone.

Treatment

Several conditions exist in which a pregnant patient requires treatment for syphilis. Along with the previously uninfected patient who now has active disease, other indications for treatment include:
1. Treatment judged to be inadequate by history, e.g., noncompliant patient with early syphilis
2. Current treatment regimen judged to be inadequate because of unsatisfactory pattern of serologic response
3. Presumed reinfection because of a rising titer
4. Previous delivery of a congenitally syphilitic infant despite presumed adequate treatment

Therapy is the same as for the nonpregnant patient. Benzathine penicillin remains the drug of choice, and serial quantitative VDRL is necessary to test for therapeutic efficacy. Table 4.4 outlines the means for differentiating and treating the various stages of syphilis.

Toxoplasmosis

Serologic tests for Toxoplasma gondii are not performed routinely in our laboratories, since intrauterine infection is quite uncommon and often difficult to determine. Between 25-33% of all women have been infected previously and are therefore immune during any re-activation of the infection. Infected newborn infants may be asymptomatic or demonstrate hydrocephaly, chorioretinitis, microphthalmia, and mental retardation. Initially asymptomatic infants may develop sequellae of the infection months to years later.

Diagnosis

The oocysts may be acquired from the maternal ingestion or handling of raw meat or exposure to feces of infected, predator cats. Toxoplasmosis should be suspected with a persistent "flu-like" illness. Lymphadenopathy may be found occasionally.

A positive serologic test (Sabin-Feldman) indicated prior infection, and any rise in titer usually represents only a reactivation of infection. A minimum 4-fold increase in titers over a 4-week period or the presence of IgM toxoplasma antibodies is necessary to diagnose a recent infection. The placenta should be examined microscopically for any oocysts.

Management

Exposure to contaminated feces of predator cats or eating raw meat should be avoided. Pregnancy termination should be offered as an option if a definitive diagnosis is made before the 20th week of gestation. Serial ultrasound examinations may be useful in assessing

Table 4.4
Treatment and Follow-up of Syphilis in Pregnancy

Syphilis Stage	Drug(s) of Choice	Alternative	Follow-up
Healthy Contact[a] or **Early** (primary, secondary, or latent 1 year)	Benzathine penicillin G 2.4 million U, IM once (half dose in each hip)	Erythromycin[b] 500 mg PO qid x 15 days	Serial VDRL titer monthly (every 3 months after delivery for 1 year
Late (more than one year's duration, benign gummatous, cardiovascular)	Benzathine penicillin G as above, weekly for 3 doses	Erythromycin as above x 30 days	CSF normal[c], no signs or symptoms of neurosyphilis: serial VDRL titer as above then every 6 months for 1-2 years. Repeat annually.
Late (neurosyphilis)	Procaine penicillin G 2.4 million U, IM (half dose in each hip) **plus** probenecid 500 mg PO qid, **both** x 10 days; followed by benzathine penicillin G (as above) weekly for 3 doses	None	CSF abnormalities or signs and symptoms of neurosyphilis[d]: follow-up as for normal CSF; also repeat LP every 3-6 months until count and protein normal
Congenital	Procaine penicillin G 50,000 U/kg IM daily x 10 days, **OR**, (only if CSF is normal) benzathine penicillin G 50,000 U/kg, IM once	None	As above, depending on stage

[a]Contact with active skin or mucous membrane lesion
[b]Poor transplacental diffusion; post-partum penicillin treatment of infant recommended
[c]CSF VDRL negative; normal protein, no pleocytosis
[d]May be asymptomatic

fetal growth and development, but a specific diagnosis is not possible by ultrasound or amniotic fluid assessment.

No specific drug therapy has been established for use during pregnancy. A 28-day course of daily sulfadiazine (4 gm) and pyrimethamine (25 mg) is perhaps most effective in halting any untoward effects, but their efficacy cannot be assessed until the infant is delivered and examined. Spiramycin is not currently available in the United States.

The pediatric staff should be notified at the time of diagnosis and well before delivery. Physical contact with an infected patient is unlikely to result in transmission of infection, so special handling precautions of an infected infant are unnecessary.

Tuberculosis

Exposure to tuberculosis is common, particularly in urban populations and in less developed countries. Up to 12.5% of gravidas may be tuberculin sensitive. A tuberculin skin test becomes positive (10 mm or more) 4-12 weeks after exposure (cell-mediated delayed sensitivity) and remains positive for a lifetime.

We routinely screen our women for tuberculosis to prevent both spread of any active or reactivated disease and fetal infection. This precaution is appropriate in populations at risk even though pregnancy, birth, puerperium and lactation do not predispose to a relapse and congenital tuberculosis is rare. A previous BCG vaccine will cause the tuberculin skin test to remain strongly positive. Guidelines for BCG administration in the non-pregnant state also apply during pregnancy.

Rubella

Approximately 15% of women of child-bearing age are not immune to rubella. Approximately one-third of all women with recently documented rubella have no symptoms, and most with symptoms have a mild 3-day rash.

Congenital defects associated with in utero rubella exposure include the development of cataracts, deafness, congenital heart disease, microcephaly, and mental retardation. Along with these birth defects, evidence for viral infection includes thrombocytopenia, hepatosplenomegaly, pneumonitis, myocarditis, and bleeding.

More than 20 kits are available for detecting rubella antibodies. Results from these kits are usually quite reliable, but sera for rubella serology should be saved for one year.

Diagnosis

When a susceptible individual is exposed to rubella, infection may develop within 2-3 weeks with antibody detectable shortly thereafter, usually coinciding with appearance of a rash. Prior test results or testing performed within 2 weeks of exosure which reveal a titer of

Evaluation after a Positive Tuberculin Skin Test

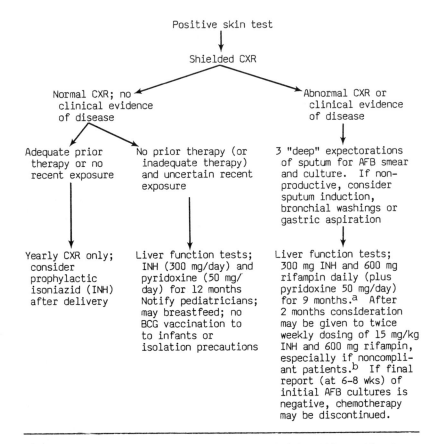

---

[a]Available as Rifamate or Rimactane/INH, containing 300 mg rifampin and 150 mg INH
[b]Usual regimen for initial treatment of all patients with uncomplicated pulmonary tuberculosis in whom drug-resistant isolates are not expected (prior treatment failure, immigrant)

$\geq$1:8 or enzyme-linked immunosorbent assay (ELISA) ratio of $\geq$1 are indicative of prior immunity. Symptoms of rubella are often inapparent but include vague flu-like illnesses for 1-5 day periods along with postauricular, cervical, and suboccipital lymphadenopathy.

A maculopapular rash usually begins on the face, spreading downward and subsequently fading in a top to bottom order.

Definitive diagnosis requires laboratory evidence of recent rubella infection. The hemagglutination inhibition antibodies, complement fixation antibodies, or ELISA values usually rise 3-5 weeks after exposure. If values drawn within 2 weeks of exposure are not indicative of immunity, the specimen should be frozen, and a second sample obtained 2-4 weeks after exposure. Both specimens should be analyzed simultaneously at the same laboratory. A 4-fold (2 dilution) increase in titer or a rising ELISA value is highly suggestive of infection.

A rubella-specific IgM antibody level may also be obtained to document any recent rubella exposure. This is particularly useful when a late serum specimen is obtained, since the rubella-specific IgM initially becomes apparent within 2 weeks after exposure and remains positive for a minimum of 4 weeks. The IgM antibody usually appears at the end of the rash, and its presence is adequate evidence for recent rubella infection. An IgM titer performed at the same laboratory as the IgG titer may also be helpful when the initial IgG titer is unexpectantly quite high (e.g., 1:1,024). Under these circumstances, the patient may be asymptomatic and was either infected recently or more likely already immune with a lingering high titer.

Prognosis

The risk of major fetal malformation varies with the gestational age at exposure with breakdown as follows:

Fetuses with major anomalies (%)	Gestational age at exposure
61	first 4 weeks
26	5-8 weeks
8	9-12 weeks
6-10	13-20 weeks

During early pregnancy, spontaneous abortion and stillbirth are 2-4 times more frequent when complicated by rubella. Impaired growth, cataracts, deafness, thrombocytopenia, and anemia may occur with exposure beyond the early organogenesis period.

There is no apparent increased risk of anomalies to fetuses exposed after the 5th month although the unborn infant may remain infected and shed the virus as a neonate. Therefore, any potentially infected infant should be isolated in the nursery.

Management

There is no specific therapy for eradicating this viral infection. Instead, supportive measures such as aspirin, fluids, and bed rest may be necessary. Therapeutic abortion should be offered as an option when clinical signs and symptoms of infection in early gestation are supported by laboratory evidence.

A rubella vaccination is indicated for those patients with antibody titers of less than 1:8. We also recommend the vaccine be given if the titer is between 1:8 and 1:16, since immunization long ago may no longer be effective. The live attenuated virus in the vaccine should be avoided for 3 months before conception or in early pregnancy. Although accidental immunization likely does little or no harm to the developing fetus and is not associated with an increased risk of anomalies, the virus has been isolated from fetal tissues and abortion specimens. The rubella vaccine should be given postpartum to nonimmune mothers, even those who are breast feeding, although passive immunity will not be transferred to the infant.

Immunizations

The diagnosis of viral infections during pregnancy is often inexact and usually by exclusion. Furthermore, pregnant patients infected by these viruses are often asymptomatic. Except for influenza, the organisms listed in Table 4.5 are associated with an increased risk of abortion or congenital and neonatal disease. The risk to the fetus is greatest during organogenesis in the first trimester. Viruses at conception may linger and affect the embryo and fetus. Signs suggesting that the newborn was infected with a virus in utero include head size abnormalities, hepatosplenomegaly, prematurity, growth retardation, hemolytic anemia, and thrombocytopenia.

Torch titers in the mother are useful only in determining whether she has had a prior exposure. When acute and convalescent sera are compared, a 4-fold increase in virus-specific IgG antibody titer is diagnostic. Virus-specific IgM titers suggest recent infection. Tests or cultures of the amniotic fluid do not provide useful information.

Accurate gestational dating is necessary, since pregnancy termination should be offered only if the diagnosis is certain and the gestational age is less than 24 weeks. These criteria are met uncommonly, however. The pediatrician should be notified at delivery about any suspected in utero viral infection, and the placenta should be sent for histologic examination as live vaccines theoretically have the ability to cross the placenta and infect the fetus; in the case of rubella, the vaccine may retain its teratogenic properties. Vaccinations using inactivated or linked viruses (influenza, hepatitis) may be used if there is a serious underlying condition. There are currently no vaccinations for coxsackie, Epstein-Barr (mononucleosis), echovirus, herpes, HIV, or cytomegalovirus infections.

Table 4.5
Recommendations for Exposure to Specific Infections during Pregnancy

	Influenza	Rubella	Tetanus-Diptheria
Maternal risk if infected	Possible increase in morbidity and mortality during epidemic of new antigenic strain	Low morbidity and mortality, not altered by pregnancy; symptomatic in only 1/3 cases	Severe morbidity; tetanus mortality 60%; diphtheria mortality 10% in respiratory cases
Fetal/ neonatal risks if inherited	Unclear; reports contradictory	Congenital rubella syndrome, severe fetal anomalies if mother infected during first trimester	Neonatal tetanus mortality 60%
Vaccine	Inactivated virus vaccine formulated according to antigentic types expected each year	Live, attenuated virus vaccine	Combined tetanus diphtheria toxoids prefer.
Fetal risk from vaccine	Unconfirmed; has been isolated in placenta	None confirmed	None confirmed
Indications for vaccination during pregnancy	Recommended only for patients with serious underlying chronic diseases	Contraindicated	Lack of primary series or no booster within past 10 years
Dose/ schedule	Adults: 0.5 ml (may depend on previous immunization)	-----	Primary: 3 doses with 2nd dose after 4-8 wks.; 3rd dose after 6 mo-1yr.; booster after 10 years
Comments	Vaccination of pregnant women left to physician's discretion	IG is not recommended for post-exposure prophylaxis, except for women who would not consider therap. abortion	Updating of immune status should be part of antepartum care

Table 4.5 (Continued)

	Varicella Zoster (Chickenpox)	Mumps	Measles
Maternal risk if infected	Low morbidity and mortality; not altered by pregnancy; pneumonia is greatest danger	Low morbidity and mortality; not altered by pregnancy	Significant morbidity; low mortality; not altered by pregnancy
Fetal/ neonatal risks, if infected	Rarely affected; increased if maternal infection shortly before delivery and direct viral contact with neonate, especially if premature (encephalomyelitis); few effects with second trimester exposure; strictures on extremities	Unlikely; questionable fibroelastosis in neonate	Risk of moderate to severe disease; association with increase in abortion rate; low birth weight; one study reports malformations
Vaccine	Zoster immune globulin or convalescent zoster plasma with 72 hr of exposure	Live, attenuated virus vaccine	Live, attenuated virus vaccine
Fetal risk from vaccine	None reported	None confirmed	None confirmed
Indications for vaccination during pregnancy	Experimental drug; no PHS recommendations for use in pregnancy	Contraindicated	Contraindicated
Dose/schedule	------	------	------

Table 4.5 (Continued)

Comments	CDC is maintaining surveillance of varicella during pregnancy	------	For immediate protection of susceptible pregnant women, use immune globulin (IG), 0.25 ml/kg; maximum dose 15 ml

Suggested Readings

Common Vaginal Infections

McLennan MT, Smith JM, McLennan CE: Diagnosis of vaginal mycosis and trichomoniasis. Obstet. Gynecol. 40:231, 1972.

Reardon EP, Noble MA, Luther ER, et al: Evaluation of a rapid method for the detection of vaginal group B streptococci in women in labor. Am. J. Obstet. Gynecol. 148:575, 1984.

Hardy PH, Nell EE, Spence MR, et al: Prevalence of six sexually transmitted disease agents among pregnant inner-city adolescents and pregnancy outcome. Lancet 2:333, 1984.

Chlamydia trachomatis infections: Policy guidelines for prevention and control. MMWR Supplement 34, August, 1985.

Gonorrhea and chlamydial infections. ACOG Tech. Bull. 89, November, 1985.

Khurana CM, Deddish PA, delMundo F: Prevalence of chlamydia trachomatis in the pregnant cervix. Obstet. Gynecol. 66:241, 1985.

Minkoff H, Mead P: An obstetric approach to the prevention of early-onset group B beta-hemolytic streptococcal sepsis. Am. J. Obstet. Gynecol. 154:973, 1986.

Morales WJ, Lim DV, Walsh AF: Prevention of neonatal group B streptococcal sepsis by the use of a rapid screening test and selective intrapartum chemoprophylaxis. Am. J. Obstet. Gynecol. 155:979, 1986.

Weisberg M: Treatment of vaginal candidiasis in pregnant women. Clin. Therap. 8:563, 1986.

Schachter J, Grossman M, Sweet RL, et al: Prospective study of perinatal transmission of chlamydia trachomatis. J. Am. Med. Assoc. 255:3374, 1986.

Gravett M, Nelson P, DeRouen T, et al: Independent associations of bacterial vaginosis and Chlamydia trachomatis infection with adverse pregnancy outcome. J. Am.. Med. Asso. 256:1899, 1986.

Urinary Tract Infection

Leveno KJ, Harris RE, Gilstrap LC, et al: Bladder versus renal bacteriuria during pregnancy: Recurrence after treatment. Am. J. Obstet. Gynecol. 139:403, 1981.

Harris RE, Gilstrap LC: Cystitis during pregnancy: A distinct clinical entity. Obstet. Gynecol. 57:578, 1981.

Lenke RR, VanDorsten JP, Schifrin BS: Pyelonephritis in pregnancy: A prospective randomized trial to prevent recurrent disease evaluating suppressive therapy with nitrofurantoin and close surveillance. Am. J. Obstet. Gynecol. 146:953, 1983.

Klein EA: Urologic problems of pregnancy. Obstet. Gynecol Surv. 39:605, 1984.

Masterton RG, Evans DC, Strike PW: Single-dose amoxycillin in the treatment of bacteriuria in pregnancy and the puerperium - a controlled clinical trial. Br. J. Obstet. Gynaecol. 92:498, 1985.

VanDorsten JP, Bannister ER: Office diagnosis of asymptomatic bacteriuria in pregnant women. Am. J. Obstet. Gynecol. 155:777, 1986.

Herpes Simplex

Corey L, Nahmias AJ, Guinan ME, et al: A trial of topical acyclovir in genital herpes simplex virus infections. N. Engl. J. Med. 306:1313, 1982.

Weinstein RA, Boyer KM, Linn ES: Isolation guidelines for obstetric patients and newborn infants. Am. J. Obstet. Gynecol. 146:353, 1983.

Jacob AJ, Epstein J, Madden DL, et al: Genital herpes infection in pregnant women near term. Obstet. Gynecol. 63:480, 1984.

Brown ZA, Vontver LA, Benedetti J, et al: Genital herpes in pregnancy: Risk factors associated with recurrences and asymptomatic viral shedding. Am. J. Obstet. Gynecol. 153:24, 1985.

Arvin AM, Hensleigh PA, Prober CG, et al: Failure of antepartum maternal cultures to predict the infant's risk of exposure to herpes simplex virus at delivery. N. Engl. J. Med. 315:796, 1986.

Harger JH, Meyer MP, Amortegui AJ: Changes in the frequency of genital herpes recurrences as a function of time. Obstet. Gynecol. 67:637, 1986.

Herpes simplex virus infections. ACOG Tech. Bull. 102, March, 1987.

Viral Hepatitis

Wong VCW, Lee AKY, Henrietta MH: Transmission of hepatitis B antigens from symptom free carrier mothers to the fetus and the infant. Br. J. Obstet. Gynaecol. 87:958, 1980.

Baker DA, Polk BF: Hepatitis B: A controllable disease. Obstet. Gynecol. 62:105, 1983.

Beasley RP, Lee G, Roan CH, et al: Prevention of perinatally transmitted hepatitis B virus infections with hepatitis B immune globulin and hepatitis B vaccine. Lancet 2:1099, 1983.

Wong VCW, Reesink HW, Reerink-Brongers EE, et al: Prevention of the HBsAg carrier state in newborn infants of mothers who are chronic carriers of HBsAg and HBeAg by administration of hepatitis-B vaccine and hepatitis-B immunoglobulin. Double-blind randomised placebo-controlled study. Lancet 1:921, 1984.

Snydman DR: Hepatitis in pregnancy. N. Engl. J. Med. 313:1398, 1985.

Wetzel AM, Kirz DS: Routine hepatitis screening in adolescent pregnancies: Is it cost effective? Am. J. Obstet. Gynecol. 156:166, 1987.

Summers PR, Biswas MK, Pastorek JG, et al: The pregnant hepatitis B carrier: Evidence favoring comprehensive antepartum screening. Obstet. gynecol. 69:701, 1987.

Acquired Immunodeficiency Syndrome

Recommendations for assisting in the prevention of perinatal transmission of human T-lymphotropic virus type III/lymphadenopathy-associated virus and acquired immunodeficiency syndrome. MMWR 34, December, 1985.

Rogers MF, Ewing EP, Warfield D, et al: Virologic studies of HTLV-III/LAV in pregnancy: Case report of a woman with AIDS. Obstet. Gynecol. 68:25, 1986.

Minkoff HL, Schwarz RH: Aids: Time for obstetricians to get involved. 68:267, 1986.

Guinan ME, Hardy A: Epidemiology of AIDS in women in the United States: 1981 through 1986. J. Am. Med. Assoc. 257:2039, 1987.

Mok JQ, DeRossi A, Ades AE, et al: Infants born to mothers seropositive for human immunodeficiency virus. Lancet 1:237, 1987.

Peckham CS, Senturia YD, Ades AE: Obstetric and perinatal consequences of human immunodeficiency virus (HIV) infection: A review.   Br. J. Obstet. Gynaecol. 94:403, 1987.

Genital Warts

Chamberlain MJ, Reynolds AL, Yeoman WB: Toxic effect of podophyllum application in pregnancy. Br. Med. J. 3:391, 1972.

Slater GE, Rumack BH, Peterson RG: Podophyllin poisoning – Systemic toxicity following cutaneous application.   Obstet. Gynecol. 52:94, 1978.

Genital human papillomavirus infections.   ACOG Tech. Bull. 105, June, 1987.

Gonorrhea

Barlow D, Phillips I: Gonorrhea in women – Diagnostic, clinical, and laboratory aspects. Lancet 1:761, 1978.

Solola AS, Ryan GM, Ling FW: Gonorrhea during the intrapartum period. Am. J. Obstet. Gynecol. 144:351, 1982.

1985 STD treatment guidelines. MMWR supplement 34, October, 1985.

Lieberman RW, Wheelock JB: The diagnosis of gonorrhea in a low-prevalence female population: Enzyme immunoassay versus culture. Obstet. Gynecol. 69:743, 1987.

Syphilis

Jones JE, Harris RE: Diagnostic evaluation of syphilis during pregnancy. Obstet. Gynecol. 54:611, 1979.

Fiumara NJ: When a pregnant woman has syphilis. Contem. Ob/Gyn 17:75, 1981.

Mascola L, Rocco P, Blount JH, et al: Congenital syphilis: Why is it still occurring? J. Am. Med. Assoc. 252:1719, 1984.

Mascola L, Pelosi R, Alexander CE: Inadequate treatment of syphilis in pregnancy. Am. J. Obstet. Gynecol. 150:945, 1984.

Toxoplasmosis

Cederquist LL, Kimball AC, Ewool LC, et al: Fetal immune response following congenital toxoplasmosis. Obstet. Gynecol. 50:200, 1977.

Stray-Pedersen B: A prospective study of acquired toxoplasmosis among 8,043 pregnant women in the Oslo area. Am. J. Obstet. Gynecol. 136:399, 1980.

Wilson CB, Remington JS: What can be done to prevent congenital toxoplasmosis? Am. J. Obstet. Gynecol. 138:357, 1980.

Frenkel JK: Congenital toxoplasmosis: Prevention or palliation? Am. J. Obstet. Gynecol. 141:359, 1981.

Desmonts G, Forestier F, Thulliez PH: Prenatal diagnosis of congenital toxoplasmosis. Lancet 1:500, 1985.

Sever JL: TORCH tests and what they mean. Am. J. Obstet. Gynecol. 152:495, 1985.

Tuberculosis

de March P: Tuberculosis and pregnancy - Five- to ten-year review of 215 patients in their fertile age. Chest 68:6, 1975.

Schaefer G, Zervoudakis IA, Fuchs FF: Pregnancy and pulmonary tuberculosis. Obstet. Gynecol. 46:706, 1977.

Covelli HD, Wilson RT: Immunologic and medical considerations in tuberculin-sensitized pregnant patients. Am. J. Obstet. Gynecol. 132:256, 1978.

Good JT, Iseman MD, Davidson PT, et al: Tuberculosis in association with pregnancy. Am. J. Obstet. Gynecol. 140:492, 1981.

Nemir RL, O'Hare D: Congenital tuberculosis: Review and diagnostic guidelines. Am. J. Dis. Child. 139:284, 1985.

Rubella

Wyll SA, Herrmann KL: Inadvertent rubella vaccination of pregnant women - Fetal risk in 215 cases. JAMA 225:1472, 1973.

Sever JL: Rubella serology: A need for improvement. Obstet. Gynecol. 56:127, 1980.

Miller E, Cradock-Watson JE, Pollock TM: Consequences of confirmed maternal rubella at successive stages of pregnancy. Lancet 2:781, 1982.

Daffos F, Grangeot-Keros L, Lebon P, et al: Prenatal diagnosis of congenital rubella. Lancet 2:1, 1984.

Enders G: Rubella antibody titers in vaccinated and nonvaccinated women and results of vaccination during pregnancy. Rev. Infect. Dis. 7:103, 1985.

Immunizations

Immunization during pregnancy. ACOG Tech. Bull. 64, May, 1982.

Brunell PA: Fetal and neonatal varicella-zoster infections. Sem. Perinatol. 7:47, 1983.

Weinstein RA, Boyer KM, Linn ES: Isolation guidelines for obstetric patients and newborn infants. Am. J. Obstet. Gynecol. 146:353, 1983.

Immunizations and chemoprophylaxis for travelers. Med. Letter 25, April, 1983.

Amstey MS, Insel RA, Pichichero ME: Neonatal passive immunization by maternal vaccination. Obstet. Gynecol. 63:105,1984.

Taina E, Hanninen P, Gronroos M: Viral infections in pregnancy. Acta Obstet. Gynecol. Scan. 64:167, 1985.

Chapter 5

Fetal Surveillance Techniques

Ultrasonography

Ultrasonography has become a highly useful tool in obstetrics. It is increasingly important for each practitioner to be cognizant of the diagnostic accuracy, range of error, and indications for its use. Some physicians have advocated routine ultrasound for all pregnant women. A recent NIH consensus conference examined this issue and concluded that there were insufficient data to demonstrate the cost effectiveness of that approach. Therefore, while universal scanning has become common in many European countries, most American obstetricians continue to reserve ultrasound for the evaluation of specific problems.

Gestational age determination, fetal growth assessment, placental localization, fetal viability evaluation, and visualization during invasive procedures remain the primary indications for obstetric ultrasound. Diagnosis of fetal malformations, biophysical assessment of uteroplacental function, placental grading, and amniotic fluid volume determination are situations in which ultrasonic monitoring has improved care of the obstetric patient.

Gestational Age Determination

Many fetal body measurements can be determined which help to assess gestational age. Measurements to be taken at certain times of gestation are shown in Table 5.1. These measurements are limited by the obstetrician's or radiologist's experience and the quality of the machine.

The earlier the gestation (26 weeks or less), the more accurate the dating parameter measurement. A biparietal diameter (BPD) or femur length (FL) measurement during the third trimester is often inaccurate. Accuracy is improved with more than one measurement with at least a 3 week interval between measurements. Confidence in dating is also improved when multiple dating parameters are measured, and averaged to yield a composite ultrasonically predicted gestational age.

137

Table 5.1
Gestational Age Determination Using Fetal Anatomic Measurements*

Time of Gestation	Growth Pattern	Accuracy (95% confidence limit)
Gestational sac 5-10 weeks	Increases 7 mm/week 2 cm at 6 weeks 5 cm at 10 weeks	Approximation
Crown-rump length (CRL) 8-14 weeks	Increases 1 cm/week 1 cm at 7 weeks 7.5 cm at 14 weeks	1 measurement: 4.7 days 3 measurements: 2.7 days
Biparietal diameter (BPD) 15-40 weeks	Increases 3 mm/week between 16-29 weeks Increases < 2 mm/week between 30-40 weeks	1 measurement: 16 weeks: 7 days 17-26 weeks: 10 days 26-28 weeks: 14 days 28 weeks: 21 days 2 measurements: Improved if at least 1 month between scan
Cerebellum diameter 15-40 weeks	Increases 1 mm/week between 15-25 weeks Increases 1.5 mm/week between 26-35 weeks Increases 2 mm/week between 35-39 weeks	Same as BPD
Head circumference 15-40 weeks	Increases 1.3 cm/week between 23-31 weeks Increases 1 cm/week between 32-40 weeks	Same as BPD
Abdominal circumference 15-40 weeks	Increases 1.1 cm/week between 14-28 weeks Increases 1 cm/week between 29-40 weeks	Same as BPD
Femur length 15-40 weeks	Increases 3 mm/week between 14-25 weeks Increases 2.3 mm/week between 26-40 weeks	Same as BPD

*See Table 1.2 for the 50th percentile values for each gestational week measurement.

The BPD is measured from the outer to inner edges of the cranium. The cranium should appear oval with no orbits being seen and the falx being midline. The thalamus and the genua of the corpus callosum should also be visualized. In contrast, the abdominal circumference (AC) and head circumference (HC) measurements are taken from outer edges and are easily performed using a tracing device.

Threatened Abortion

Visible milestones include seeing the gestational sac as early as 5 weeks, embryo at 7 weeks, and fetal heart motion at 8 weeks. A blighted ovum or missed abortion is to be suspected if there is no growth or a regression of the sac over a 2-week period, and no fetal limb or heart motion is seen after the 8th week. However, if fetal cardiac activity is observed, the probability of continued pregnancy without abortion is greater than 94%.

Fetal Malformation

As more ultrasound examinations are being performed on pregnant women, a higher percentage of fetal malformations is detected in utero than was in the past. A fetal malformation may be seen for the first time during a genetic amniocentesis or may be suggested by polyhydramnios or oligohydramnios. Visualization of internal structures (cerebral ventricles, heart valves, stomach, bowel, kidneys, bladder) along with surface anatomy (head, neck, limbs, spine, male genitalia) is possible with currently available equipment. Under most circumstances, it is best to have the ultrasound examination repeated by a highly experienced ultrasonographer for purposes of documentation, education, and additional useful information.

Any fetal malformation should be brought to the attention of a geneticist or teratologist. It is preferred that the ultrasound exam be performed in the presence of a staff neonatologist or pediatrician who can then provide further counseling to the parents, plan for the care of an infant deemed salvageable, and discussion of the case with the appropriate pediatric surgical service.

Uterine Size Less than Dates

Conditions to consider include inaccurate dates, intrauterine growth retardation (IUGR), oligohydramnios (secondary to IUGR, infection, ruptured membranes, renal anomaly), and fetal descent into the pelvis. Delayed fetal growth should initially be suspected when bimanual examination shows uterine size less than estimated gestational age.

Suspected IUGR

The following findings on ultrasound examination may strengthen the suspicion of IUGR or permit a more accurate dating of the pregnancy.

BPD
1. The BPD measurement is frequently not helpful and can even be misleading in the evaluation of IUGR because fetal head growth is usually relatively spared in this condition.
2. Consider microcephaly if the body size is appropriate but BPD and HC measurements are small.
3. Look for a low profile or late flattening pattern of the skull.
4. Rare if BPD more than 50th percentile for gestational age.

Oligohydramnios
1. A normal amount of amniotic fluid is unusual in pregnancies complicated by IUGR.
2. Failure to observe a pocket of fluid measuring at least 2 cm (in perpendicular dimensions) suggests moderately severe oligohydramnios which is present in approximately 40% of cases of IUGR.

Femur Length
1. Useful if dating uncertain, or if dwarfism or IUGR suspected.
2. Need to compare with BPD measurements.
3. After 22 weeks the femur length to abdominal circumference ratio (FL:AC) equals 0.22 + .02 in normally growing fetuses. A FL:AC > 0.24 is suggestive of IUGR.
4. IUGR unlikely if distal femoral epiphysis seen.

Head Circumference/Abdominal Circumference (HC/AC)
1. Ratio decreases with gestational age.
2. Equivalent measurements at 36 weeks.
3. Asymmetric IUGR in 60% of cases if HC/AC value is in 95th percentile for age.
4. Failure of the AC to increase by at least 10 mm over a 14 day period is highly suggestive of IUGR.

Estimated Fetal Weight
1. Acccurate gestational age determination necessary.
2. Measurements of the BPD or FL and AC necessary for weight prediction using published tables.
3. Often inaccurate if there is oligohydramnios, fetal malpresentation, maternal obesity, or fetal weight more than 2,500 gms.

Uterine Size Greater than Dates

Conditions to consider include inaccurate dates, large for gestational age (LGA) fetus, multifetal gestation, polyhydramnios, pelvic mass (uterine fibroid, ovarian tumor), and hydatidaform mole. These abnormalities may be suspected during the bimanual examination and can be confirmed by ultrasound.

Multifetal Gestation

1. Can usually see two sacs in the first trimester, but 20% of twins seen on early ultrasound "vanish" or spontaneously regress.
2. 3% of twins may be monoamnionic (1 sac only) which is associated with a 50% perinatal mortality from umbilical cord entanglement, twin-twin transfusion, birth trauma, and congenital anomalies.
3. After 24 weeks, repeat scans every 3-6 weeks to search for:
   a. BPD growth (BPD growth curve for normally growing twins is essentially the same as for singletons)
   b. Intertwin growth discordance. Difference in BPD's (more than 5 mm), HC's (more than 5%), AC's (more than 5%), or weights (more than 15%). Prognosis is poorer if discordance present at ages of less than 28 weeks
   c. Twin-twin transfusion (differences in amniotic fluid volume, fetal size, fetal heart rate)
   d. Anomalies
   e. Fetal well-being (biophysical profile - breathing patterns, limb motion, muscle tone, amniotic fluid volume, placental morphology).

Third Trimester Bleeding

Placenta Previa
1. Placental location and margin may be seen in almost all pregnancies.
2. Posterior placenta may be shadowed by fetus.
3. Exact location of cervix is necessary but may be difficult to localize.
4. Need post-void film if full maternal bladder (may "push" anterior placenta toward cervix).
5. Placenta "migrates" during pregnancy due to development of lower uterine segment, consequently most second trimester previas disappear by term.
6. If central previa found during the first half of pregnancy, repeat scan indicated in third trimester.

Placental Abruption
1. Very difficult to diagnose using ultrasound.
2. May appear as an echo free area behind a convex placenta, a thick placenta because of a heterogeneous clot, or a rounded elevation of the membranes by the clot.
3. Sonolucent area behind the placenta is usually a normal second trimester artifact.
4. A thickened placenta (more than 5 cm) may also result from diabetes, Rh isoimmunization, syphilis, nonimmune fetal hydrops, chorioangioma, or trophoblastic disease.

Additional Uses

1. Before, during, or after special procedures: amniocentesis, cervical cerclage, intrauterine fetal transfusion, external version of breech fetus, locating the fetal heart during heart rate monitoring, locating placenta before cesarean section
2. Fetal presentation determination
3. Intrauterine fetal demise (IUFD) diagnosis: no fetal heart or limb motion, collapsed cranium
4. Localizing fetal heart rate and other body parts during the delivery of a second twin
5. Visualizing intrauterine cavity when delayed postpartum or postabortal hemorrhage

Other Techniques

Doppler Flow Studies

The combination of real-time sonography and Doppler equipment permits noninvasive measurement of fetal blood flow especially in the umbilical vessels and descending aorta. Sonographic localization of the umbilical vein in the fetal abdomen is followed by Doppler measurement of blood velocity. This technique may improve the accuracy of prediction of physiologic reserve, especially for high risk pregnancies such as those with hypertension or fetal growth retardation in which chronic uteroplacental insufficiency is likely.

It has been suggested that diminished umbilical vein blood flow may be an earlier diagnostic sign of fetal distress than fetal heart rate testing. Doppler flow studies may provide a reflection of the amount of oxygenation, since the fetus, placenta, and umbilical cord have a great capacity to shunt blood to vital organ centers (brain, heart, adrenals) during periods of relative hypoxia. Whether reduced umbilical blood flow is the cause or result of chronic fetal hypoxia is unclear at this time. Large clinical trials are being performed which may clarify and broaden the role of Doppler ultrasound.

M-Mode Echocardiography

Imaging the fetal heart and directly measuring parameters that reflect myocardial contractility and ventricular size has become possible with the introduction of real-time-directed M-mode echocardiography. The capability to noninvasively assess fetal cardiac disorders can provide information which is useful in prenatal counseling, appropriate management of the pregnancy and delivery, and planning of specialized neonatal care. This technique also has potential use in the prenatal investigation of fetal cardiac spatial anatomy and cardiac rhythm disturbances.

The standard echocardiogram involves viewing the long axis, great vessel short axis, forechamber, and aortic arch. Fetal cardiac failure can be detected, its etiology can be better clarified, and serious cardiac malformations may be excluded. Dysrhythmias may also be better characterized. Adjacent structural abnormalities which may impinge on cardiac function include intrathoracic or abdominal cavity anomalies.

Magnetic Resonance Imaging (MRI)

When certain anomalies of the fetus are first suspected by ultrasound, better clarification may be possible using more expensive magnetic resonance imaging. No ionizing radiation is involved, and this imaging technique is particularly well-suited for characterization of dilated, fluid-filled structures (such as hydrocephalus). It also reveals maternal pelvic organs quite clearly and makes possible measurements of the bony pelvis.

Antepartum Fetal Heart Rate Testing (AFHRT)

Antepartum fetal heart rate testing (AFHRT) has gained popularity in the biophysical assessment of fetal well-being. Data are readily interpretable and provide timely results. The nonstress test (NST) indirectly measures the intactness of the fetal autonomic and central nervous systems during fetal movement, while the contraction stress test (CST) reflects the respiratory and nutritive reserve (baro- and chemoreceptors) of the fetoplacental unit during the stress of spontaneous or oxytocin-induced uterine contractions.

These tests are quite useful in predicting fetal well-being and favorable results are associated with a low probability of antepartum stillbirth. Any suspicious result requires a thorough clinical reassessment, good clinical judgment, and additional tests. In general, the nonstress test has replaced the contraction stress test as the initial AFHRT test. It is a test of convenience, however, and any suspicious finding requires a CST (or repeat NST later that day).

Nonstress tests are performed during outpatient visits in most cases. The tests may be performed any time during the third trimester (28 weeks or more) with the realization that an abnormal result requires further follow-up. Most tests are usually not performed until 32 weeks or later.

Indications

These tests are indicated when there is any suggestion of uteroplacental insufficiency. Pregnancies complicated by postdates, discordant twins, diabetes, suspected IUGR, preeclampsia, chronic hypertension, collagen vascular disease, or documented decreased fetal activity are associated with chronic uteroplacental insufficiency and would benefit the most from fetal heart rate testing.

Technique

NST
1. Place patient in a semi-Fowler's or lateral tilt position.
2. Determine the fetal heart rate variability and reactivity in association with fetal and uterine activity.
3. Instruct mother on fetal movement recording.
4. Monitor mother's blood pressure periodically for any signs of supine hypotension.

CST
1. Same as steps 1-4 above.
2. If no spontaneous uterine or fetal activity, ask the mother to gently stimulate a nipple to promote uterine contractions. In the unlikely event that nipple stimulation does not result in an adequate contraction pattern, begin oxytocin infusion (0.5-1.0 mu/min.). The dose should be doubled every 15 minutes until there are at least three contractions every 10 minutes, repetitive late decelerations, or hypertonic uterine contractions.
3. After discontinuing the oxytocin, observe for any persisting uterine contractions.

Interpretation

Standard definitions of a nonreactive or reactive NST and a negative, suspicious, or positive CST are shown in Table 5.2. Considerations during test interpretation should include physician experience, prolonged maternal supine positioning, maternal obesity, polyhydramnios, excess fetal activity or inactivity, physiologic fetal rest period (up to 1 hour), abnormal fetal lie, and instability of any underlying complication(s).

Nonstress test results are not influenced by maternal weight, smoking, caffeinated beverages, drugs, ambulation, or a recent meal. Instead, FHR reactivity is more dependent on the fetal activity pattern and the primary underlying complication. Preterm rupture of the membranes does not affect the reliability of NST results.

If the NST result is reactive, it is generally safe to wait up to 1 week before repeating the test again. However, any acute change in the underlying antepartum complication (such as worsening diabetes), an umbilical cord accident, or a placental abruption may lead to fetal compromise and distress. Decelerations of the fetal heart rate during an NST may relate to maternal position or hypotension. If decelerations are repetitive despite a reactive result, a CST is indicated because there may be a cord complication or fetal hypoxia.

A CST is contraindicated in the presence of an unknown or vertical uterine scar, prior premature labor, multifetal gestation, third trimester bleeding, or preterm rupture of the fetal membranes. If a NST is nonreactive and a CST is contraindicated, a fetal biophysical profile (fetal breathing movement, fetal muscle tone and motion of

Table 5.2
Interpretation of Antepartum Fetal Heart Rate Tests

NST

Reactive:	2 or more adequate FHR accelerations (15 beats/min above baseline, lasting 15 sec or more) during a 20-40 minute period
Nonreactive:	0-1 adequate accelerations during the 20-40 minute test period

CST

Negative:	No late deceleration with uterine contractions (3 in 10 minutes)
Suspicious:	Any decelerations which are not persistent (coincident with 50% or less of adequate contractions)
Positive:	Repetitive late decelerations (coincident with more than 50% of contractions)

---

limbs, amniotic fluid volume, and placental morphology) using ultrasonography should be performed.

A positive CST is more likely to be a truly worrisome finding if a nonreactive pattern was present, a deceleration was seen on a prior NST, the fetus remains inactive, or the obstetric or medical condition is deteriorating. A cesarean section is not absolutely necessary after a positive CST, however. Depending on the clinical condition, a trial of labor with early amniotomy and internal monitoring may be performed.

Management of NST Results

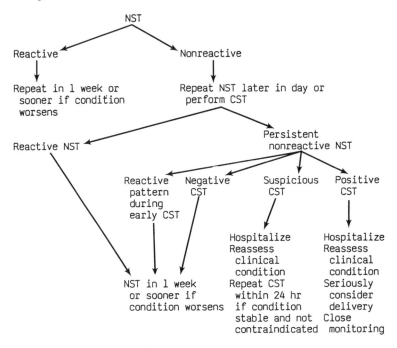

Biophysical Profile

The earliest attempts to evaluate fetal well-being by ultrasound were based on anatomic considerations. The vitality of the fetal central nervous system may be inferred indirectly from observing heart rate testing or movement charting. Because antepartum fetal heart rate testing methods are time consuming and may yield false positive results, obstetricians have included ultrasound visualizations in certain circumstances to more thoroughly evaluate fetal status. Evaluation of fetal activity, muscle tone, and breathing movements also provides useful information in predicting fetal well-being. However, each parameter considered alone may be falsely positive, and results may be unreliable in predicting fetal outcome.

In recent years, a "biophysical profile" has been proposed where results of the nonstress test and observation of fetal activity, fetal muscle tone, fetal breathing, and amniotic fluid volume are combined into one composite score (Table 5.3). This profile has been used to evaluate high risk pregnancies of many different pathologic processes.

Table 5.3
Technique and Interpretation of Biophysical Profile Scoring

Biophysical variable	Normal (score = 2)	Abnormal (score = 0)
Fetal breathing movements	One or more episodes of $\geq$30 sec in 30 min	Absent or no episode of $\geq$30 sec in 30 min
Gross body movements	Three or more discrete body/limb movements in 30 min (episodes of active continuous movement considered as single movement)	Two or less episodes of body/limb movements in 30 min
Fetal tone	One or more episodes of active extension with return to flexion of fetal limb(s) or trunk; opening and closing of hand considered normal tone	Either slow extension with return to partial flexion or movement of limb in full extension or absent fetal movement
Reactive fetal heart rate	Two or more episodes of acceleration of $\geq$15 bpm and of $\geq$15 sec associated with fetal movement in 20 min	Less than 2 episodes of acceleration of fetal heart rate or acceleration of $\geq$15 bpm in 40 min
Qualitative amniotic fluid	One or more pockets of fluid measuring $\geq$1 cm in two perpendicular planes	Either no pockets or <1 cm in two perpendicular planes

Along with performing a nonstress test, the main body of the profile takes approximately 30 minutes to perform.

Each of the biophysical variables is given a score of 2 if normal or 0 if abnormal. Therefore, the maximum achievable score is 10 and the low score is 0. Studies have shown that this profile provides a better prediction of fetal distress in labor, 5 minute Apgar scores, and perinatal mortality than any other method used alone. If the composite score is 8-10, the test is repeated in one week unless the patient has passed her estimated date of confinement or is an insulin-dependent diabetic. There is no indication for promptly delivering the infant if the score is 8 or greater. If the composite score is 4-6, there is cause for concern and delivery should be considered if fetal pulmonary maturity is demonstrated. A score of 0-2 would require the pregnancy to be delivered without delay.

Fetal Movement Charting

The monitoring of fetal activity is a convenient surveillance technique in high risk pregnancies. Although not a direct test of placental function, it serves as a signal of impending fetal jeopardy and possibly death. The maternal awareness of a recent decrease or loss of propulsive fetal motion has been traditionally regarded as a warning sign, especially in pregnancies complicated by hypertension, diabetes, or Rh isoimmunization, where chronic uteroplacental insufficiency is suspected.

Technique

Many testing schemes have been developed, and the superiority of any one method has not been established. Described below is a daily fetal movement charting (DFMC) technique which we have found to be practical:
1. Fetal movement charting may begin at any time during the second half of pregnancy; however, it is particularly useful during the third trimester.
2. The patient is asked to rest, preferably in a lateral recumbent position, in a quiet room for at least one convenient hour each day. The counting may be discontinued in 30 minutes if the fetus is found to be active.
3. Strong or propulsive fetal movements ("rollovers," "balling up," "kicks" not "flutters" or "hiccups") are recorded on a standard fetal movement chart. Clusters of movements should be counted as one.
4. The patient should also be asked to report any concern about a significant decrease in the total number or loss in strength of fetal movements.
5. A new chart should be given to the patient with each return visit, and the previous chart should be placed on the prenatal record.

Interpretation

The average fetus is perceived to move 24 times/hr and this rate does not decrease significantly near term. As long as the fetus is healthy, this average does not decrease markedly despite the presence of an antepartum complication. It should be remembered that each fetus has its own activity pattern, and no two pregnancies are alike in that respect.

A fetus is considered to be active if four or more movements are perceived per hour. Fetal inactivity is defined on our services as being three or fewer movements perceived per hour for 2 consecutive hours. An excessively active fetus (40 movements or more per hour over a prolonged period) is not an unfavorable sign.

Advantages and Limitations

Advantages
1. No cost
2. No technician or physician time
3. Data collection anywhere
4. Daily monitoring
5. Decreases use of more expensive or time-consuming tests in borderline cases
6. Encourages patient to rest on her side, perhaps improving uteroplacental circulation
7. Improves patient awareness of her unborn baby

Limitations
1. Like other antepartum fetal tests, limited in predicting acute fetal distress and most major malformations (acute fetal distress from umbilical cord accidents or acute placental complications may not be detected)
2. Occasional difficulty in differentiating between a normal but "slow" fetus and a fetus in jeopardy
3. Patient subjectivity in perceiving motions, especially if weak "flutters"
4. Continued patient cooperation (best if patient understands physician concerns, understands the technique, and is seen regularly by the same doctor)
5. Can be confusing with multifetal gestation

Workup of Fetal Inactivity

The decision to intervene in the presence of fetal inactivity should not be based on fetal movement studies alone. Any patient complaining of a decrease in fetal activity on routine questioning should be instructed to chart fetal movements. Documented fetal inactivity or a patient concern about a lack of movement (despite hearing a heart rate) should be a warning sign which requires further investigation, although a seemingly slow but continuously moving fetus may be doing quite well.

Real-Time Ultrasonography
Determine viability
Observe for fetal cardiac
 motion, lower limb and
 trunk motion, breathing
 activity
Search for a malformation
Characterize placental
 morphology and amniotic
 fluid volume

Vigorous movement seen
Reassure
Assess patient's ability to perceive
 fetal motion using ultrasound
Resume fetal movement counting
 and other fetal assessment methods
Lack of vigorous movement seen
Further testing by:
 Antepartum fetal heart rate testing
 Biophysical profile measurements
No movement
Offer uterine evacuation

Fetal Lung Maturity Testing

Respiratory distress syndrome (RDS) or more specifically, hyaline membrane disease is found in approximately 15% of infants with birth weights of 2,500 gms or less. Prevention of RDS may be unavoidable if the patient is delivered prematurely for obstetric or medical complications. Respiratory insufficiency results from a deficiency of surfactant, a material which provides a stable surface tension within the alveolar spaces. Alveolar surface tension is diminished with insufficient surfactant, and the lungs collapse during expiration.

Surfactant is composed of phospholipid compounds which include phosphatidylcholine (lecithin), phosphatidylglycerol (PG), phosphatidylinositol (PI), and disaturated phosphatidyl choline (DSPC). Although other amniotic fluid tests have been used in predicting fetal maturity, the most reliable means for quantitating pulmonary surfactant involves a measurement of these abundant phospholipids.

Lecithin/Sphingomyelin Ratio (L/S)

This ratio is the most standardized and widely used determination for fetal pulmonary maturity. The assay technique is critical, since variations in centrifugation, activation of thin layer plates for separation of the phospholipids, moisture, and densitometer precision may all adversely affect test results.

As a general rule, a mature L/S ratio (greater than or equal to 2:1) is predictive of fetal lung maturity (and lack of subsequent neonatal RDS) in 97% of cases. A ratio 1.5-1.9 is associated with respiratory distress in half of infants, while a value below 1.5 is associated with a 73% risk of respiratory distress. These percentages vary depending on the laboratory and clinical criteria used in the interpretation of respiratory distress.

Phosphatidylglycerol (PG)

This phospholipid may be measured despite presence of meconium or blood in the amniotic fluid or after preterm rupture of the amniotic membranes. PG determinations are useful and reliable in conjunction with L/S measurements in pregnancies with Rh isoimmunization or diabetes in which a "mature" L/S ratio may be erroneous and misleading. Phosphatidylglycerol does not generally appear until 35 weeks gestation but increases in quantity until the 40th week.

Other Fetal Lung Maturity Tests

Although less often reported, other reliable tests to assess fetal lung maturity include:
1. Optical density measurements at 650 mu (a value 0.15 or greater correlates with a mature L/S ratio)
2. Microviscosity from the high relative lipid concentration of amniotic fluid

3. "Shake" test or foam stability index (FSI) to determine whether pulmonary surfactant is present in adequate amounts to generate a stable foam in the present of ethanol
4. Measurement of disaturated phosphatidylcholine (DSPC)
5. Monoclonal antibody testing against phosphatidylglycerol.

In all tests, a positive test result is reassuring, but falsely decreased or "immature" results are frequently reported. An advantage of certain of these tests is the ability to perform the test without sophisticated laboratory facilities.

General Recommendations

The L/S ratio has been widely recognized in the "gold standard" for assessing fetal lung maturity. If there is a condition which would suggest a falsely mature L/S value or if the test result is borderline, the L/S ratio alone may be inadequate. Two conditions commonly associated with a falsely mature L/S ratio are diabetes mellitus and Rh isoimmunization, in which there is a relative fetal hyperinsulinemia. The use of another test would be recommended in such cases.

These test results should be used only as additional information when preterm pregnancy intervention or repeat cesarean section is anticipated. A laboratory result should not replace good clinical judgment when management of a high risk pregnancy is considered.

Examination of the infant is essential to assess the predictability of the amniotic fluid test. Evidence of respiratory distress in the neonate includes definite clinical findings (nasal flaring, grunting, and tachypnea), chest x-ray findings (reticulogranular pattern), and need for supplemental oxygen therapy.

Suggested Readings

Ultrasonography

Crane JP, Tomich PG, Kopta M: Ultrasonic growth patterns in normal and discordant twins. Obstet. Gynecol. 55:678, 1980.

Diagnostic ultrasound in obstetrics and gynecology. ACOG Tech. Bull. 63, October, 1981.

Shepard MJ, Richards VA, Berkowitz RL, et al: An evaluation of two equations for predicting fetal weight by ultrasound. Am. J. Obstet. Gynecol. 142:47, 1982.

Hill LM, Breckle R, Wolfgram KR: An ultrasonic view of the developing fetus. Obstet. Gynecol. Surv. 38:375, 1983.

Birnholz JC: Determination of fetal sex. N. Engl. J. Med. 309:942, 1983.

Bartolucci L, Hill WC, Katz M, et al: Ultrasonography in preterm labor. Am. J. Obstet. Gynecol. 149:52, 1984.

DeVore GR, Siassi B, Platt LD: Fetal echocardiography IV. M-mode assessment of ventricular size and contractility during the second and third trimesters of pregnancy in the normal fetus. Am. J. Obstet. Gynecol. 150:981, 1984.

Bakketeig LS, Jacobsen G, Brodtkorb CH, et al: Randomised controlled trial of ultrasonographic screening in pregnancy. Lancet 2:207, 1984.

Campbell S, Warsof SL, Little D, et al: Routine ultrasound screening for the prediction of gestational age. Obstet Gynecol. 65:613, 1985.

Fleischer A, Schulman H, Farmakides G, et al: Umbilical artery velocity waveforms and intrauterine growth retardation. Am. J. Obstet. Gynecol. 151:502, 1985.

Maulik D, Nanda NC, Moodley S, et al: Application of Doppler echocardiography in the assessment of fetal cardiac disease. Am. J. Obstet. Gynecol. 151:951, 1985.

Weinreb JC, Lowe T, Cohen JM, et al: Human fetal anatomy: MR imaging. Radiology 157:715, 1985.

Vintzileos AM, Campbell WA, Nochimson DJ, et al: Antenatal evaluation and management of ultrasonically detected fetal anomalies. Obstet. Gynecol. 69:640, 1987.

Ahram J, Feinstein SJ, DePhillips H: Survey of ultrasound training in obstetrics and gynecology residency training programs in the United States. Obstet. Gynecol. 70:405, 1987.

Goldstein I, Reece EA, Pilu G, et al: Cerebellar measurements with ultrasonography in the evaluation of fetal growth and development. Am. J. Obstet. Gynecol. 156:1065, 1987.

Antepartum Fetal Heart Rate Testing

Phelan JP: The nonstress test: A review of 3,000 tests. Am. J. Obstet. Gynecol. 139:7, 1981.

Rayburn WF, Motley ME, Zuspan FP: Conditions affecting nonstress test results. Obstet. Gynecol. 59:490, 1982.

Antepartum fetal surveillance. ACOG Tech. Bull. 107, August, 1987.

Platt LD, Paul RH, Phelan J, et al: Fifteen years of experience with antepartum fetal testing. Am. J. Obstet. Gynecol. 156:1509, 1987.

Smith CV, Nguyen HN, Kovacs B, et al: Fetal death following antepartum fetal heart rate testing: A review of 65 cases. Obstet. Gynecol. 70:18, 1987.

Keegan KA, Helm DA, Porto M, et al: A prospective evaluation of nipple stimulation techniques for contraction stress testing. Am. J. Obstet. Gynecol. 157:121, 1987.

Devoe LD,, Morrison J, Martin J, et al: A prospective comparative study of the extended nonstress test and the nipple stimulation contraction stress test. Am. J. Obstet. Gynecol. 157:531, 1987.

Gagnon R, Campbell K, Hunse C, et al: Patterns of human fetal heart rate accelerations from 26 weeks to term. Am. J. Obstet. Gynecol. 157:743, 1987.

Thacker SB, Berkelman RL: Assessing the diagnostic accuracy and efficacy of selected antepartum fetal surveillance techniques. Obstet. Gynecol. Surv. 41:121, 1986.

Biophysical Profile

Manning FA, Platt LD, Sipos L: Antepartum fetal evaluation: Development of a fetal biophysical profile. Am. J. Obstet. Gynecol. 136:787, 1980.

Platt LD, Eglinton GS, Sipos L, et al: Further experience with the fetal biophysical profile. Obstet. Gynecol. 61:480, 1983.

Manning FA, Lange IR, Morrison I, et al: Fetal biophysical profile score and the nonstress test: A comparative trial. Obstet. Gynecol. 64:326, 1984.

Manning FA, Morrison I, Lange IR, et al: Fetal assessment based on fetal biophysical profile scoring: Experience in 12,620 referred high-risk pregnancies I. Perinatal mortality by frequency and etiology. Am. J. Obstet. Gynecol. 151:343, 1985.

Devoe LD, Searle N, Searle J, et al: Computer-assisted assessment of the fetal biophysical profile. Am. J. Obstet. Gynecol. 153:317, 1985.

Benacerraf BR, Frigoletto FD: Fetal respiratory movements: Only part of the biophysical profile. Obstet. Gynecol. 67:556, 1986.

Vintzileos AM, Gaffney SE, Salinger LM, et al: The relationships among the fetal biophysical profile, umbilical cord pH, and Apgar scores. Am. J. Obstet. Gynecol. 157:627, 1987.

Fetal Movement Charting

Birnholz JC, Stephens JC, Faria M: Fetal movement patterns: A possible means of defining neurologic developmental milestones in utero. Am. J. Roentgenol. 130:537, 1978.

Patrick J, Campbell K, Carmichael L, et al: Patterns of gross fetal body movements over 24-hour observation intervals during the last 10 weeks of pregnancy. Am. J. Obstet. Gynecol. 142:363, 1982.

Dierker LJ, Pillay SK, Sorokin Y, et al: Active and quiet periods in the preterm and term fetus. Obstet. Gynecol. 60:65, 1982.

Nyholm HC, Hansen T, Neldam S: Fetal activity acceleration during early labor. Acta Obstet. Gynecol. Scand. 62:131, 1983.

Rayburn WF: Clinical implications from monitoring fetal activity. Am. J. Obstet. Gynecol. 144:967, 1982.

Natale R, Nasello C, Turliuk R: The relationship between movements and accelerations in fetal heart rate at twenty-four to thirty-two weeks' gestation. Am. J. Obstet. Gynecol. 148:591, 1984.

Sadovsky E, Rabinowitz R, Freeman A, et al: The relationship between fetal heart rate accelerations, fetal movements, and uterine contractions. Am. J. Obstet. Gynecol. 149:187, 1984.

Fetal Lung Maturity Tests

Grannum PAT, Berkowitz RL, Hobbins JC: The ultrasonic changes in the maturing placenta and their relation to fetal pulmonic maturity. Am. J. Obstet. Gynecol. 133:915, 1979.

Dombroski RA, Mackenna J, Brame RG: Comparison of amniotic fluid lung maturity profiles in paired vaginal and amniocentesis specimens. Am. J. Obstet. Gynecol. 140:461, 1981.

Whittle MJ, Wilson AI, Whitfield CF: Amniotic fluid phosphatidylglycerol and the lecithin/sphingomyelin ratio in the assessment of fetal lung maturity. Br. J. Obstet. Gynaecol. 89:727, 1982.

Sher G, Statland BE: Assessment of fetal pulmonary maturity by the lumadex foam stability index test. Obstet. Gynecol. 61:444, 1983.

Garite RJ, Yabusaki KK, Moberg LJ, et al: A new rapid slide agglutination test for amniotic fluid phosphatidylglycerol: Laboratory and clinical correlation. Am. J. Obstet. Gynecol. 147:681, 1983.

Lipshitz J, Whybrew WD, Anderson GD: Comparison of the lumadex-foam stability index test, lecithin: Sphingomyelin ratio, and simple shake test for fetal lung maturity. Obstet. Gynecol. 63:349, 1984.

Kazzi GM, Gross TL, Sokol RJ, et al: Noninvasive prediction of hyaline membrane disease: An optimized classification of sonographic placental maturation. Am. J. Obstet. Gynecol. 152:213, 1985.

Herbert WNP, Chapman JF: Clinical and economic considerations associated with testing for fetal lung maturity. Am. J. Obstet. Gynecol. 155:820, 1986.

Benoit J, Merrill S, Rundell C, et al: Amniostat-FLM: An initial clinical trial with both vaginal pool and amniocentesis samples. Am. J. Obstet. Gynecol. 154:65, 1986.

Weiner SH, Weinstein L: Fetal pulmonary maturity and antenatal diagnosis of respiratory distress syndrome. Obstet. Gynecol. Surv. 42:75, 1987.

Chapter 6

Fetal Disorders

Intrauterine Growth Retardation

An infant whose birth weight is less than the 10th percentile for that gestational age is classified as having undergone intrauterine growth retardation (IUGR). Depending on the population, 5-7% of infants will be growth retarded. These infants are at increased risk for perinatal mortality, intrapartum asphyxia, neonatal acidosis, hypoglycemia, hypocalcemia, and polycythemia. The lower the birth weight percentile, the greater the likelihood of fetal jeopardy.

Growth retardation may be characterized further as being symmetric (early onset, usually from a genetic or teratogenic insult) or asymmetric (late onset, usually due to inadequate fetal nutrition either from inadequate maternal nutrition or diseases limiting placental transfer of nutrients). Infants with asymmetric growth retardation usually have a good long-term prognosis if neonatal complications are adequately controlled, while the prognosis for a symmetrical growth retarded infant is more guarded. The etiologies of intrauterine growth retardation are many and are listed in Table 6.1.

Diagnois

Clinical Evaluation

Only one third of fetuses with IUGR are diagnosed antenatally and in only one-half of these is the diagnosis of a truly growth retarded infant confirmed at delivery. Most truly growth retarded infants have an obstetric, medical, nutritional, or social history suggesting a risk for IUGR. A knowledge of gestational age and a high index of suspicion are necessary. Abnormally low fundal height measurements have a 86% sensitivity and 90% specificity for IUGR.

Table 6.1
Etiology of Intrauterine Growth Retardation

Chromosomal
  Turner's syndrome
  Trisomy 21, 18, 13

Drugs
  Heroin
  Methadone
  Cocaine
  Pentazocine
  Alcohol
  Coumadin
  Phenytoin
  Trimethadione

Infection
  TORCH agents

Antepartum hemorrhage
  Abruptio placenta
  Placenta previa

Maternal vascular disease
  Toxemia
  Chronic hypertension
  Renal disease
  Cyanotic heart disease
  Severe diabetes (Class D, F, R)
  Collagen vascular disease

Tobacco
  Carbon monoxide
  Nicotine
  Cyanide
  Others

Maternal anemia
  Iron deficiency
  Folate deficiency
  Hemoglobinopathy

Other
  Maternal malnutrition
  Multifetal gestation

Ultrasound Evaluation

The development of ultrasound has enhanced our ability to evaluate potentially growth retarded infants. While many tests have been proposed, the optimal diagnostic accuracy is obtained by employing multiple ultrasound parameters.

The BPD tends to remain in the same growth percentile (less than the 25th, 25th to 75th, more than the 75th). A drop from the upper groups to the lower group is highly suggestive of growth retardation. The diagnosis is unlikely if the BPD is greater than the 50th percentile. Failure of BPD to increase over 3 weeks is a poor prognostic sign. Additionally a delay in biparietal diameter, head circumference, or abdominal circumference, in relation to the cerebellar diameter is indicative of IUGR.

A head/abdominal circumference ratio greater than the 95th percentile suggests asymmetric IUGR. Campbell has reported that this parameter is falsely negative in 29% of cases, however. An increase in the abdominal circumference of < 10 mm over a 14 day period may be the most sensitive ultrasound marker for IUGR. Frequently, this is associated with a femur length/abdominal circumference ratio greater than the 95th percentile (i.e. ≥ 0.24).

An ultrasonographically estimated fetal weight less than the 10th percentile is suggestive of IUGR. The diagnostic accuracy of this test is reported to be within 100 gms per kilogram of body weight.

Most pregnancies complicated by IUGR have subjectively decreased quantities of amniotic fluid. Although most demonstrate pockets > 1-2 cm in perpendicular dimensions, those pregnancies with pockets of 1 cm or less are commonly found to have an IUGR fetus.

Amniotic Fluid Maturity Evaluation

Many IUGR infants demonstrate accelerated pulmonary maturity. This fact is useful in differentiating the truly IUGR from the misdated pregnancy. The finding of an amniotic fluid Foam Stability Index Value 47 in the presence of a BPD $\leq$ 8.5 cm has been reported to have an 84% sensitivity and near 100% specificity for the diagnosis of IUGR. Similarly, others have found an 80% sensitivity for the diagnosis of IUGR when phosphatidylglycerol is detected and the BPD measures $\leq$ 8.7 cm.

Management

Accurate Gestational Dating

Medical Treatment
1. Frequent reclining on left side
2. Stop smoking
3. High protein (100 gm/day) and 2,500 calories/day diet
4. Fetal movement charting in combination with either NSTs, CSTs, or biophysical profiles
5. Ultrasound every 3-4 weeks until third trimester, then as often as weekly for biophysical assessment
6. Weekly or semi-weekly exams after 32 weeks

Appropriately Timed Interruption of Pregnancy
1. Several investigators advocate delivery when the fetus is mature (L/S > 2 or PG present). This form of management removes the fetus from the hostile environment but increases the risk of cesarean section. Others feel that the benefit of this routine approach has not been documented, and as cesarean section rates are high, the patient should instead be followed until there is a favorable Bishop cervix score, another abnormal fetal test result, or a worsening of the maternal disease.
2. Delivery of the immature fetus despite an absence of risk factors or a stable underlying condition is indicated only if antepartum tests are clearly abnormal. If a test result is suspicious, the test should be repeated within 24 hours as long as the condition is stable. Corticosteroid therapy should be given if delivery is anticipated at or before 32 weeks or if the L/S ratio is known to be less than 2:1.

Careful Management of Labor
1. Lateral position of mother
2. Oxygen to mother by face mask or nasal prongs as necessary
3. Electronic fetal monitoring; selective scalp pH sampling

4. Be prepared to perform a cesarean section if fetal distress becomes apparent
5. Avoid meconium aspiration
6. Early clamping of umbilical cord since these fetuses tend to be hemoconcentrated
7. Obtain umbilical cord blood pH

Meticulous Neonatal Care
1. Pediatrician in attendance
2. Orderly resuscitation
3. Diagnosis and management of hypoglycemia, hypocalcemia, hyperviscosity, meconium aspiration, renal problems (if asphyxia), altered thermoregulation
4. Proper nutrition to improve growth
5. Suspect genetic or infectious etiology if no other known risk factors
6. Placenta for careful histologic examination

Fetal Macrosomia

A large or macrosomic fetus is defined as having a weight in the upper 10th percentile which at term would be greater than 4,000 gms. Clinical suspicion is necessary, since the disorder is associated with diabetes mellitus, Rh isoimmunization, and postdates. Mechanical difficulties and trauma during labor and delivery should be anticipated.

Diagnosis

Estimation of fetal weight is dependent on clinical and ultrasound examinations. A weekly bimanual pelvic examination is useful within 2 weeks of the estimated due date to determine the presenting part, condition of the cervix, size of the pelvis, and estimation of fetal weight. Ultrasound examinations are limited in diagnosing fetal macrosomia but may permit measuring the biparietal diameter, abdominal circumference, and amniotic fluid volume. A BPD greater than 10.5 cm at term is strongly suggestive of fetal macrosomia or hydrocephaly, and a chest-biparietal diameter difference of 1.4 cm or greater is suggestive of macrosomia in a fetus of a diabetic mother.

Management

When fetal macrosomia is suspected, documentation on the prenatal record is necessary. Glucose tolerance testing is indicated, and the maternal blood type and antibody screen should be determined. If fetal macrosomia is suspected in any gestational onset diabetic, low dose NPH insulin therapy (10-20 units daily) along with dietary surveillance is recommended as early in gestation as possible in an attempt to ultimately lower the birth weight. Other conditions associated with fetal macrosomia include large parents, a space-occupying anomaly, alpha thalassemia, nonimmune fetal hydrops, postdates, and Beckwith's syndrome. Many infants are healthy and have no obvious reason for their large size.

Macrosomia is associated with an increased risk of a traumatic vaginal delivery such as shoulder dystocia, brachial plexus injury, clavicular fracture, and maternal soft tissue injury. Any pregnancy in which macrosomia is suspected should be monitored closely during labor using internal uterine catheters and fetal heart rate monitoring devices. A cesarean section is recommended if there is either early evidence of fetal distress, failure to adequately descend during labor, or breech presentation. A cesarean section without a trial of labor is permissible for macrosomia alone if an especially large fetus $\geq 4,500$ gms) is anticipated or the fetus is 4,000 gms or more in a diabetic pregnancy.

If a macrosomic infant is delivered, it should be followed carefully for evidence of hypoglycemia. A maternal serum hemoglobin A_1C should be drawn to screen for any previous glucose intolerance.

Nonimmune Fetal Hydrops

Fetal hydrops not related to maternal isoimmunization was first described in 1943. Until recently, most cases were not detected until birth. The widespread application of diagnostic ultrasound has resulted in a dramatic upsurge in the antenatal diagnosis.

While the prognosis is usually poor (90% perinatal mortality) because of the resultant pulmonary hypoplasia or coexisting major anomalies, some infants may be salvaged with careful antepartum evaluation and meticulous neonatal care. A variety of conditions involving the fetus, placenta, or mother may cause nonimmune fetal hydrops and are listed in Table 6.2.

Antepartum Evaluation

1. Accurate gestational dating
2. Blood type and antibody screen
3. Serologic test for syphilis (RPR)
4. TORCH screen
5. Kleihauer-Betke test
6. Glucose tolerance test
7. Ultrasonography, serial (chest, abdomen, neck, surface anatomy, placenta, umbilical cord)
8. Fetal echocardiography
9. Nonstress tests
10. Fetal movement charting
11. Amniotic fluid for karyotype (if delivery not anticipated soon)

Table 6.2
Etiology of Nonimmune Fetal Hydrops

Fetal
  Hematologic
    Fetomaternal or twin-twin
    transfusion, alpha thalassemia,
    G6PD deficiency
  Multiple gestation with
    parasitic fetus
  Cardiovascular
    Congenital heart disease,
    (ASD, VSD, hypoplastic
    left heart, pulmonary
    insufficiency, intracardiac
    tumor, Ebstein's anomaly,
    subaortic stenosis, tricuspid
    valvular dysplasia, tetralogy
    of Fallot), premature
    closure of foramen ovale
    Tachyarrhythmias (SVT,
    atrial flutter, heart block)
    Fibroelastosis
    Myocarditis
  Pulmonary
    Cystic adenomatoid malformation
    Pulmonary lymphangiectasia
    Pulmonary hypoplasia

  Renal
    Congenital nephrosis
    Renal dysplasia
    Renal vein thrombosis
  Intrauterine infection
    TORCH
    Leptospirosis
    Congenital hepatitis
    Chagas disease
  Miscellaneous
    Meconium peritonitis
    Fetal neuroblastoma
    Small bowel volvulus
    Disseminated intravascular
    coagulation
    Chromosomal-trisomy 18, trisomy
    21, Turner's syndrome, XX/XY
    mosaicism
    Achondroplasia
    Tuberous sclerosis
    Storage disease
    Polycystic ovaries
    Sacral teratoma

Placental
  Umbilical vein thrombosis
  Chorionic vein thrombosis
  Chorioangioma

Maternal
  Diabetes mellitus

Idiopathic

Therapy

Before 25 Weeks
Treat any fetal cardiac dysrhythmia and offer termination if chromosome
abnormality or potentially life-threatening anomaly

Between 25-32 Weeks
Treat any fetal cardiac dysrhythmia
Deliver if progressive hydrops (pleural or pericardial effusions)
Corticosteroid therapy may enhance fetal lung maturity

After 32 Weeks
Deliver if fetal lung maturity, fetal distress, or evidence of progressive hydrops

Before Delivery
Notify pediatrician well in advance
Expect birth asphyxia, anemia, and hypovolemia and plan on resuscitation
Pediatrician at delivery and pediatric surgery notified

Infant Evaluation

1. Complete blood count with differential
2. Platelet count
3. Blood type and Coomb's test
4. VDRL
5. Serum IgM level
6. Liver function tests
7. Renal function tests
8. ECG, echocardiography
9. Chromosomal analysis
10. Cultures (bacterial and viral), TORCH screen
11. X-rays (chest, abdomen, long bones, skull)
12. Diagnostic paracentesis and/or thoracentesis
13. Placental anatomy and histologic evaluation
14. Retrieve blood samples before any transfusions
15. Placental histologic examination

Polyhydramnios

Polyhydramnios is defined as 2 liters or more of amniotic fluid. The incidence is reported to be 0.4% of all pregnancies. The etiology is variable, but conditions are similar to those contributing to non-immune fetal hydrops (Table 6.2). Diabetes, isoimmunization, multifetal gestation, and congenital abnormalities are frequently present. A definite cause is not identifiable in more than half of cases, but most malformations associated with polyhydramnios may be visualized prenatally.

An acute rather than chronic onset has a less favorable prognosis. The more severe the polyhydramnios, the higher the probability of a fetal anomaly. Clinical suspicion is best confirmed by ultrasound examination. Methods to evaluate the mother and fetus are listed in Table 6.3.

Antepartum Management

1. If etiology unknown, wait until L/S 2 or greater. Concentrations of amniotic fluid PG, creatinine, etc. may be falsely low
2. Amniocentesis if immature fetus and maternal respiratory compromise, premature labor, or marked uterine distension. Using

a 18-gauge spinal needle or Angiocath and an intravenous infusion set connected to a sterile container (example: thoracentesis bottle) on the floor, 500-2,000/ml of fluid should be removed slowly at approximately 500 ml/hr. A higher gauge needle should not be used, because drainage may be too slow or the system may become clotted. Fetal heart rate monitoring should be performed after the amniocentesis (immediately if blood is retrieved). The amniocentesis may be repeated in usually 1-3 weeks depending on the patient's symptoms

3. Bedrest in lateral recumbent position
4. Frequent examinations are necessary for maternal abdominal circumference, and fundal height measurements, weight, and signs of congestive heart failure
5. High protein diet
6. Frequent maternal serum electrolyte and protein determinations
7. Weekly ultrasound examinations to assess fetal growth and activity, placental morphology and integrity, and amniotic fluid volume
8. Biophysical profiles, fetal movement charting and fetal heart rate testing, even though each is often of limited value (poorly discernible tracing, cord compression patterns)
9. If premature labor, may use tocolytic agent if etiology remains unknown, or immature L/S ratio and no other complications
10. Deliver if mature fetus or evidence of fetal distress
11. Notify pediatricians after diagnosis confirmed and before anticipated delivery

Table 6.3
Evaluation of Polyhydramnios

Maternal
 Accurate pregnancy dating
 1-hr post glucola serum glucose (3-hr GTT if abnormal)
 Irregular antibody screen
 Observe weight gain and fundal height

Fetal
 Ultrasound to rule out multifetal gestation and to examine:
  Head size: BPD, ventricle-to-hemisphere ratio
  Fetal swallowing and neck width
  Chest cavity (heart rate, valve action, pericardial effusion, pleural effusion, breathing motion)
  Abdomen (masses, bowel atresia, wall masses, kidney outline, bladder filling)
  Skeletal system (especially vertebral volumne and limb length)
  Placental characteristics
  Echocardiography (?)

Intrapartum Management

1. Baseline complete blood count, fibrinogen, platelets
2. Type and screen mother's blood
3. Slowly remove 500-1,000 ml of fluid before any induction; carefully control release during labor
4. Watch for placental abruption, umbilical cord prolapse, and postpartum uterine atony
5. Placenta to be sent to pathology
6. Cesarean section if any fetal distress during monitoring, fetal malpresentation, suspected space occupying anomaly, or placental abruption

Fetal Hydrocephaly

The diagnosis of fetal hydrocepnaly should be considered during ultrasound examination when the lateral ventricles are found to extend more than halfway from the midline falx to the lateral skull table. Since asynclitisim can frequently distort the relationship between various intracranial structures, the diagnosis of hydrocephalus should always be confirmed by a highly experienced obstetric ultrasonographer. Occasionally the diagnosis is made before the late second trimester when the option of therapeutic abortion is still a viable alternative. However, most often hydrocephalus is an unanticipated finding during an ultrasound exam in the latter half of the pregnancy.

Infants with other congenital abnormalities (approximately 85% with intracranial or extracranial anomalies such as open spinal defects), a shift of the midline intracranial structures, a cerebral mantel thickness less than 10 mm, an expansion of the hydrocephaly, or a head circumference greater than 50 cm have a poorer prognosis for normal neurological function. An absolute correlation between ultrasound findings and subsequent neurological function is presently unclear. If any cerebral mantel remains and no other abnormalities are present, the fetus should probably not be subjected to a destructive procedure to facilitate vaginal delivery. Attempts at intrauterine ventricular amniotic shunts have been attempted but have met with quite limited success.

Etiology

A neonatologist and neurosurgeon should be notified before delivery. The route of delivery and initial evaluation of the newborn infant are important for subsequent therapy and genetic counseling. Treatment and prognosis of hydrocephalus are based on whether it is a communicating or noncommunicating lesion (Table 6.4). After initial antepartum evaluation, pregnancy is followed by ultrasonic examination to determine whether the hydrocephalus is progressive or stable.

Table 6.4
Etiology of Fetal Hydrocephaly

Noncommunicating	Communicating
Aqueductal stenosis (may be x-linked recessive) Dandy-Walker cyst Intracranial mass	Arnold-Chiari malformation Encephalocele Inflammation of the leptomeninges Lissencephaly Congenital absence of arachnoid granulations Choroid plexus papilloma

Proposed Management

Antepartum Evaluation
Baseline ultrasound measurements
Establish etiology if possible
Rule out other anomalies (especially spina bifida),
Scan weekly to look for stable or progressive
  ventriculomegaly

Stable Hydrocephalus
Serial scans comparing
 lateral ventricle width
 with hemispheric width
Conservative management
 with cesarean section as
 route of delivery

Progressive Hydrocephalus
Evidence on weekly ultrasound
 exams of further ventricular
 enlargement and cerebral
 cortex compression
Consider intrauterine CAT scan
 or MRI

Pulmonary   No pulmonary
maturity   maturity

Cesarean   Continue until
section   pulmonary
                   maturity if
                   very immature

No remaining mantel, HC 50 cm
 or more, or asymmetric
 ventriculomegaly

Vaginal delivery
Avoid decompression (will
 distort anatomy on autopsy
 exam later)
If unsatisfactory labor or
 obstruction, decompress head
 in utero. Use an 18-gauge
 spinal needle or intrauterine
 transfusion needle by
 transvaginal rather than
 transabdominal approach if
 possible

Fetal Dysrhythmias

Up to 15% of fetuses have some form of cardiac dysrhythmia in utero. Diligent evaluation of the maternal history, physical examination, and fetus is required to identify a fetus whose cardiovascular function is severely compromised. Most infants with dysrhythmias (especially irregular or "skipped" heart beats) do well in the antepartum and intrapartum periods. These dysrhythmias often convert to a normal sinus rhythm at or shortly after birth. Fetal heart rate abnormalities may be classified into three major groups: tachycardia, bradycardia, and irregular.

Tachycardia
(Atrial tachycardia, atrial flutter, complete AV block, supraventricular tachycardia)

Evaluation
1. 2-dimensional echocardiography (to characterize the dysrhythmia, outline any structural defect, or thoracic anomaly)
2. Serial ultrasound examinations (search for polyhydramnios, hydrops, body size dimensions)
3. Fetal well-being tests (movement charting, ultrasound visualization, NST if FHR less than 200)
4. Careful neonatal observation and evaluation

Management
1. Notify pediatricians
2. Maternal digoxin therapy - usually 0.25 mg daily if evidence for fetal heart rate failure (verapamil or propranolol if no response to digoxin)
3. Early delivery if fetal lung maturity or fetal distress and no response to maternal medication
4. If conversion successful await spontaneous labor with close monitoring during stress of uterine contractions
5. A vaginal delivery may initiate a vagal response and convert the rapid heart rate to a more normal rate

Bradycardia
(Complete heart block)

Evaluation
1. 2-dimensional echocardiography (if severe or associated with failure)
2. Serial ultrasonography (search for polyhydramnios, hydrops, delayed fetal growth, pericardial effusion)
3. Other fetal well-being tests (movement charting, ultrasound visualization)
4. Amniocentesis for fetal karyotype if delivery not imminent
5. Serum ANA (many mothers will have or develop systemic lupus erythematosis)

Management
1. Notify pediatricians
2. Maternal isoproterenol or digoxin therapy if fetal immaturity and signs of distress or heart failure
3. Early delivery if fetal lung maturity or evidence of distress, and no response to medication
4. Careful neonatal observation and evaluation (may require a pacemaker)

Irregular

(Premature atrial contractions, premature ventricular flutters)

Evaluation and management same as for bradycardia

Recurrence Risks of Malformations

Between 2-4% of all infants will have one or more major malformations at birth. Most are usually not life-threatening but may be disfiguring. The diagnosis is usually made at delivery after an unremarkable prenatal course. Often malformations are isolated and multifactorial in nature, but a karyotype is recommended if there is any question of diagnosis, if an associated chromosomal abnormality is suspected, or if more than one major anomaly is found.

Along with a discussion of treatment alternatives by the infant's physician, new parents should be reassured that the risk of recurrence is low. Recurrence risks of certain malformations are listed in Table 6.5. Ultrasound examinations are recommended in subsequent pregnancies, although many of these malformations cannot be visualized. A genetic amniocentesis is unnecessary, however, unless the previous infant had a known chromosomal abnormality, an open neural tube defect, or a detectable inborn error of metabolism.

The Stillborn Infant and Repeated Abortion

The stillbirth rate in the United States is presently 9-10 per 1,000 live births. When possible, it is important to determine the etiology of the fetal death. Of equal importance is protection of the maternal and family psychosocial health.

Historical and physical data may provide important clues. Helpful information includes accurate gestational dating, medical or obstetrical complications, maternal blood type and antibody screen, exposures to noxious agents (drugs, x-rays, infection), outcome of prior pregnancies, ethnic background and genetic histories, and occupations. A total body x-ray or photograph of the fetus is recommended for the permanent records, patient, and referring physician. An instamatic camera may be found in most labor and delivery room areas.

Table 6.5
Recurrence Risk of Specific Malformations

Cleft lip with or without cleft palate	
One affected child	4%
Two affected children	9%
One affected parent	4%
One affected parent and one affected child	17%
Cleft palate only	
One affected child	2%
Two affected children	10%
One affected parent	6%
One affected parent and one affected child	15%
Open neural tube defects	
One affected child	2-4%
Two affected children	10-12%
Hydrocephaly	1%
Congenital heart disease	
Ventricular septal defect	5%
Atrial septal defect	3%
Patent ductus arteriosus	4%
Pulmonic stenosis	3%
Aortic stenosis	2%
Tetralogy of Fallot	3%
Transposition of great vessels	2%
Coarctation of aorta	2%
Clubfoot	3%
Congenital hip dislocation	4-5%
Pyloric stenosis	
One affected child	3%
Mother affected	16%
Father affected	5%
Hypospadias	3%
Abdominal muscle deficiency (prune belly)	1%
Arthrogryposis (congenital contractures)	5-15%
Craniosynostosis	1-2%
Renal agenesis, bilateral (Potter)	1-3%
VATER syndrome	10%

The placenta, cord, and membranes should be examined carefully. A description of the gross appearance of the placenta should be recorded in the medical record. The placenta should be prepared in formalin and appropriate clinical information gathered (including the patient's registration number and delivery date) before being sent to pathology.

An autopsy of the products of conception is recommended for detailed analysis of morphology and visceral and somatic growth. Along with an assessment of craniofacial proportions and specific organs, body measurements should include the crown-rump, crown-heel, arm, leg, and foot lengths. Specimens of preferably amniotic fluid or fresh tissues (skin, amnion, or liver) should be placed in a sterile container with saline and sent promptly to a genetics laboratory for karyotyping. Chromosomal aberrations are associated with 50-60% of all first trimester abortions and 5-10% of stillbirths. Autosomal trisomy comprises approximately 50% of chromosomally abnormal abortuses and monosomy X occurs in 25% of abortuses. Parental karyotyping is suggested for cases of repeated pregnancy loss for determination of any blanced translocation or inversion.

Testing of the mother should also include a Kleihauer-Betke test (at the time of stillbirth), thyroid function test, glucose tolerance screening; renal function test, serum immunologic testing (ANA, anticardiolipin antibody, lupus anticoagulant, partial thromboplastin), and toxoplasmosis titer. The cervix should be cultured for listeria, chlamydia and mycoplasma. A hysterosalpingogram after menses have resumed may provide helpful information

With repeated first trimester pregnancy losses, the patient should be instructed on basal body temperature charting, and a serum progesterone should be obtained after conception is suspected. If test results do not provide a possible explanation for repeated abortion, an immunologic etiology should be considered. The likelihood of another spontaneous abortion is at least 25% and may be greater if the abortus had a normal chromosomal complement or if there had been no other live-born offspring.

Grief Response

An immediate and delayed grief response by the expectant parents is natural and to be anticipated. Half of all women who experience a perinatal death will require prolonged psychiatric treatment or hospitalization within the next 12 months. The psychological effects of the father are less well documented. Facilitation of the grieving process at the time of death and during the first 6 postpartum weeks may decrease the incidence of psychiatric complications.

The mother should be warned that she may have difficulty with normal daily functions such as eating and sleeping. She may also dream about the infant and imagine that she hears or sees the infant. These are not signs of significant psychiatric illness, rather they are a part of the normal grieving process.

The couple should be counseled that in American society, most adults do not perceive the death of a fetus or child less than 1 year of age in the same light as they would perceive the death of an older person. Therefore, acquaintances may make what appear to be somewhat callous comments such as, "Don't worry about it. You can have another one."

It should also be explained to parents that other children frequently experience sibling rivalry toward the unborn fetus and may consider the death to be a result of these feelings. Therefore, the death should be discussed specifically with the children, and they should be told that they had nothing to do with its cause.

If the family decides to name the infant or have a funeral, these actions may provide reality and closure to the event. However, the family should not be forced to take these actions if they do not feel they are appropriate. Bodies sent to pathology or for autopsy are usually cremated. It is frequently helpful to see the family for a prolonged interview approximately one month postpartum to assess their adaptation to the loss, discuss any autopsy or placental findings, and describe implications for future pregnancies. Pregnancy should not be encouraged until the couple is ready both psychologically and emotionally.

Suggested Readings

Intrauterine Growth Retardation

Sholl JS, Woo D, Rubin JM, et al: Intrauterine growth retardation risk detection for fetuses of unknown gestational age. Am. J. Obstet. Gynecol. 144:709, 1982.

Neilsen JP, Munjanja SP, Whitfield CR: Screening for small for dates fetuses: A controlled trial. Br. Med. J. 289:1179, 1984.

Seeds JW: Impaired fetal growth: Ultrasonic evaluation and clinical management. Obstet. Gynecol. 64:577, 1984.

Erskine RLA, Ritchie JWK: Umbilical artery blood flow characteristics in normal and growth-retarded fetuses. Br. J. Obstet. Gynaecol. 92:605, 1985.

Divon MY, Chamberlain PF, Sipos L, et al: Identification of the small for gestational age fetus with the use of gestational age-independent indices of fetal growth. Am. J. Obstet. Gynecol. 155:1197, 1986.

Villar J, Belizan JM: The evaluation of the methods used in the diagnosis of intrauterine growth retardation. Obstet. Gynecol. Surv. 41:187, 1986.

Fetal Macrosomia

Golditch IM, Kirkman K: The large fetus management and outcome. Obstet. Gynecol. 52:26, 1978.

Parks DG, Ziel HK: Macrosomia: A proposed indication for primary cesarean section. Obstet. Gynecol. 55:407, 1978.

Modanlou HD, Dorchester WL, Thorosian A, et al: Macrosomia - maternal, fetal, and neonatal implications. Obstet. Gynecol. 55:420, 1980.

Elliott JP, Garite TJ, Freeman RK, et al: Ultrasonic prediction of fetal macrosomia in diabetic patients. Obstet. Gynecol. 60:159, 1982.

Ounsted M, Moar VA, Scott AA: Risk factors associated with small-for-dates and large-for-dates infants. Br. J. Obstet. Gynaecol. 92:226, 1985.

Langer O, Brustman L, Anyaegbunam A, et al: The significance of one abnormal glucose tolerance test value on adverse outcome in pregnancy. Am. J. Obstet. Gynecol. 157:758, 1987.

Leikin EL, Jenkins JH, Pomerantz GA, et al: Abnormal glucose screening tests in pregnancy: A risk factor for fetal macrosomia. Obstet. Gynecol. 69:570, 1987.

Bochner CJ, Medearis AL, Williams J, et al: Early third-trimester ultrasound screening in gestational diabetes to determine the risk of macrosomia and labor dystocia at term. Am. J. Obstet. Gynecol. 157:703, 1987.

Nonimmune Fetal Hydrops

Holzgreve W. Curry CJR, Golbus MS, et al: Investigation of nonimmune hydrops fetalis. Am. J. Obstet. Gynecol. 150:805, 1984.

Mostoufi-Zadeh M, Weiss LM, Driscoll SG: Nonimmune hydrops fetalis: A challenge in perinatal pathology. Human Pathol. 16:785, 1985.

Landrum BG, Johnson DE, Ferrara B, et al: Hydrops fetalis and chromosomal trisomies. Am. J. Obstet. Gynecol. 154:1114, 1986.

Castillo RA, Devoe LD, Hadi HA, et al: Nonimmune hydrops fetalis: Clinical experience and factors related to a poor outcome. Am. J. Obstet. Gynecol. 155:812, 1986.

Watson J, Campbell S: Antenatal evaluation and management in nonimmune hydrops fetalis. Obstet. Gynecol. 67:589, 1986.

Gough JD, Keeling JW, Castle B, et al: The obstetric management of non-immunological hydrops. Br. J. Obstet. Gynaecol. 93:226, 1986.

Hsieh FJ, Chang FM, Ko TM, et al: Percutaneous ultrasound-guided fetal blood sampling in the management of nonimmune hydrops fetalis. Am. J. Obstet. Gynecol. 157:44, 1987.

Polyhydramnios

Alexander ES, Spitz HB, Clark RA: Sonography of polyhydramnios. Am. J. Roentgenol. 138:343, 1982.

Quinlan RW, Cruz AC, Martin M: Hydramnios: Ultrasound diagnosis and its impact on perinatal management and pregnancy outcome. Am. J. Obstet. Gynecol. 145:306, 1983.

Flowers WK: Hydramnios and gastrointestinal atresias: A review. Obstet. Gynecol. Surv. 38:685, 1983.

Chamberlain PF, Manning FA, Morrison I, et al: Ultrasound evaluation of amniotic fluid volume II. The relationship of increased amniotic fluid volume to perinatal outcome. Am. J. Obstet. Gynecol. 150:250, 1984.

Hill LM, Breckle R, Thomas ML, et al: Polyhydramnios: Ultrasonically detected prevalence and neonatal outcome. Obstet. Gynecol. 69:21, 1987.

Cardwell MS: Polyhydramnios: A review. Obstet. Gynecol. Surv. 42:612, 1987.

Fetal Hydrocephaly

Chervenak FA, Berkowitz RL, Romero R, et al: The diagnosis of fetal hydrocephalus. Am. J. Obstet. Gynecol. 147:703, 1983.

Vintzileos AM, Ingardia CJ, Nochimson DJ: Congenital hydrocephalus: A review and protocol for perinatal management. Obstet. Gynecol. 62:539, 1983.

Chervenak FA, Ment LR, McClure M, et al: Outcome of fetal ventriculomegaly. Lancet 2:234, 1984.

Chervenak FA, Berkowitz RL, Tortora M, et al: The management of fetal hydrocephalus. Am. J. Obstet. Gynecol. 151:933, 1985.

Michejda M, Queenan JT, McCullough D: Present status of intrauterine treatment of hydrocephalus and its future. Am. J. Obstet. Gynecol. 155:873, 1986.

Fetal Dysrhythmias

Young BK, Katz M, Klein SA: Intrapartum fetal cardiac arrhythmias. Obstet. Gynecol. 54:427, 1979.

Shenker L: Fetal cardiac arrhythmias. Obstet. Gynecol. Surv. 34:561, 1979.

Hawrylyshyn PA, Miskin M, Gilbert BW, et al: The role of echocardiography in fetal cardiac arrhythmias. Am. J. Obstet. Gynecol. 141:223, 1981.

DeVore GR, Donnerstein RL, Kleinman CS, et al: Fetal echocardiography I. Normal anatomy as determined by real-time directed M-mode ultrasound. Am. J. Obstet. Gynecol. 144:249, 1982.

Kleinman CS, Donnerstein RL, DeVore GR, et al: Fetal echocardiography for evaluation of in utero congestive heart failure. N. Engl. J. Med. 306:568, 1982.

Crawford D, Chapman M, Allan L: The assessment of persistent bradycardia in prenatal life. Br. J. Obstet. Gynaecol. 92:941, 1985.

Recurrence Risks of Malformations

Kirk EP, Wah RM: Obstetric management of the fetus with omphalocele or gastroschisis: A review and report of one hundred twelve cases. Am. J. Obstet. Gynecol. 146:512, 1983.

Kalter H, Warkany J: Congenital malformations – Etiologic factors and their role in prevention (first of two parts). N. Engl. J. Med. 308:424, 1983.

Kalter H, Warkany J: Congenital malformations (second of two parts). N. Engl. J. Med. 308:491, 1983.

Hobbins JC, Romero R, Grannum P, et al: Antenatal diagnosis of renal anomalies with ultrasound I. Obstructive uropathy. Am. J. Obstet. Gynecol. 148:868, 1984.

Rubin JD, Ferencz C: Subsequent pregnancy in mothers of infants with congenital heart disease. Pediatrics 76:371, 1985.

Main DM, Mennuti MT: Neural tube defects: Issues in prenatal diagnosis and counselling. Obstet. Gynecol. 67:1, 1986.

Chervenak FA, Isaacson G, Mahoney MJ: Advances in the diagnosis of fetal defects. N. Engl. J. Med. 315:325, 1986.

Allan LD, Crawford DC, Chita SK, et al: Prenatal screening for congenital heart disease. Br. Med. J. 292:1717, 1986.

The Stillborn Infant and Repeated Abortion

Fay RA: Feto-maternal haemorrhage as a cause of fetal morbidity and mortality. Br. J. Obstet. Gynaecol. 90:443, 1983.

Harger JH, Archer DF, Marchese SG, et al: Etiology of recurrent pregnancy losses and outcome of subsequent pregnancies. Obstet. Gynecol. 62:574, 1983.

Royston D, Geoghegan F: Amniotic fluid infection with intact membranes in relation to stillborns. Obstet. Gynecol. 65:745, 1985.

Rayburn W, Sander C, Barr M, et al: The stillborn fetus: Placental histologic examination in determining a cause. Obstet. Gynecol. 65:637, 1985.

Grief related to perinatal death. ACOG Tech. Bull. 86, April, 1985.

Kiely JL, Paneth N, Susser M, et al: Fetal death during labor: An epidemiologic indicator of level of obstetric care. Am. J. Obstet. Gynecol. 153:721, 1985.

McDonough PG: Repeated first-trimester pregnancy loss: Evaluation and management. Am. J. Obstet. Gynecol. 153:1, 1985.

Diagnosis and management of fetal death. ACOG Tech. Bull. 98, November, 1986.

Scott JR, Rote NS, Branch DW: Immunologic aspects of recurrent abortion and fetal death. Obstet. Gynecol. 70:645, 1987.

Woods J, Esposito J (eds.): Pregnancy Loss: Medical Therapeutic and Practical Considerations. Baltimore, Williams & Wilkins, 1987.

Chapter 7

Special Procedures

Genetic Amniocentesis and Genetic Counseling

Certain genetic disorders may be diagnosed by prenatal genetic counseling and prenatal diagnostic testing. Because of the widespread availability of amniotic fluid sampling in early pregnancy, most test results are normal which is reassuring. Primary indications for genetic amniocenteses include:

Maternal age 35 years or older
Prior infant with inborn error of metabolism
Prior infant or family history of open neural tube defects
Mother known to be a carrier of an X-linked disorder
Prior infant with a chromosomal disorder
History of habitual abortion

Any patient 35 years or older is at increased risk of delivering an infant with a chromosomal abnormality (Table 7.1). The likelihood of there being a cytogenetic abnormality at age 35 is 1/180 which exceeds the generally accepted risk of fetal demise or abortion following amniocentesis (less than 1/200). The rates of fetal loss, low birth weight, neonatal complications, and birth defects are not more common in the amniocentesis group than in the control group. We do not routinely perform a genetic amniocentesis for a woman less than 35 years old because of overutilization of our laboratories, procedure risk being greater than the benefit from the test result, and cost effectiveness.

A patient who previously delivered a child with an autosomal or sex chromosomal trisomy has a 1-2% risk of delivering another affected child in each subsequent pregnancy. A parent may be found to be a balanced translocation carrier after karyotype evaluation for infertility or repeated pregnancy wastage. These individuals usually appear normal but may produce offspring with chromosomal translocations. The risk of delivering an infant with a unbalanced translocation depends on the chromosomal site involved. The risk for D/G is 4% if the father is a carrier, for D/G is 9-11% if the mother is a carrier, and for G/G is 100%.

X-linked recessive disorders such as Duchenne muscular dystrophy and hemophilia are transmitted by women carrying the trait to 50% of

175

Table 7.1
Chromosomal Abnormalities per 1000 Live Births*

Maternal Age	Down's Syndrome alone	Any chromosomal abnormality
30	0.9-1.2	2.6
31	0.9-1.3	2.6
32	1.1-1.5	3.1
33	1.4-1.9	3.5
34	1.9-2.4	4.1
35	2.5-3.9	5.6
36	3.2-5.0	6.7
37	4.1-6.4	8.1
38	5.2-8.1	9.5
39	6.6-10.5	12.4
40	8.5-13.7	15.8
41	10.8-17.9	20.5
42	13.8-23.4	25.5
43	17.6-30.6	32.6
44	22.5-40.0	41.8
45	28.7-52.3	53.7
46	36.6-68.3	68.9
47	46.6-89.3	89.1
48	59.5-116.8	115.0
49	75.8-152.7	149.3

*From Hook, E.B., Obstet. Gynecol. 58:282, 1981.

male fetuses but will not be transmitted to female fetuses. Therefore, an amniocentesis for karyotype determination is useful to determine the sex of the fetus. An absolute diagnosis can only be made by sampling fetal blood using fetoscopy, placental aspiration, or umbilical cord blood sampling.

An amniocentesis may be useful in diagnosing a fetus affected by sickle cell anemia or thalassemia. Genetic mapping by DNA fragment analysis of retrieved amniotic fluid cells has been helpful in determining mutations of the beta-globulin chain. Using restriction endonuclease enzymes, the DNA may be more discernible at specific base sequences to determine any abnormal fragments.

Most biochemical genetic disorders are autosomal recessive in inheritance. The recurrence risk for a couple delivering another affected infant is 25% in these situations. However, a few biochemical disorders (osteogenesis imperfecta) are autosomal dominant with a recurrence risk of 50%. More than 100 of these biochemical disorders may be diagnosed prenatally by analysis of cellular enzymes responsible for mucopolysaccharide, carbohydrate, lipid, or amino acid metabolic derangements. Table 7.2 lists commonly described biochemical disorders and whether tests are available for prenatal detection.

Table 7.2
Biochemical Disorders that May Be Detected Prenatally

Disorder	Biochemical Defect	Prenatal Diagnosis
Adrenogenital syndromes	Metabolites of 11-, 17-, or 21-steroid hydroxylase	Yes
Chronic granulo-matous disease	Granulocyte NBT reduction	Yes
Cystic fibrosis	MUGR reactive, proteases	Possible
Ehlers-Danlos syndrome, type IV	Unknown (lack of type III collagen)	Possible
Fabry disease**	Ceramidetrihexoside galactosidase	Yes
Galactosemia	Galactose-1-phosphate uridyl transferase	Yes
Gaucher disease	Glucocerebrosidase	Yes
Glycogen storage disease, type III (Pompe disease)	-1, 4-Glucosidase	Yes
Hemoglobinopathies	Synthesis of abnormal hemoglobin	Yes
Hemophilia A*	Factor VIII deficiency	Yes
Hemophilia B	Factor IX deficiency	Yes
Hunter syndrome	-L-Iduronic acid-2 sulfatase	Yes
Hurler syndrome	-L-Iduronidase	Yes
Hyperammonemia, type II	Ornithine carbamyltransferase	Probable
Hyperthyroidism	Unknown (reverse tri-iodothyronine level)	Possible
Hypothyroidism	Multiple (reverse tri-iodothyronine level)	Possible
Krabbe disease	Galactocerebroside B-galactosidase	Yes
Maple syrup urine disease	Branched-chain ketoacid decarboxylase	Yes

Table 7.2 (Continued)

Disorder	Biochemical Defect	Prenatal Diagnosis
Menkes disease	Unknown (copper incorporation)	Probable (in some cases)
Niemann-Pick disease	Sphingomyelinase	Yes
Phenylketonuria	Phenylalanine hydroxylase	Possible
Placental sulfatase deficiency**	Placental sulfatase	Yes
Porphyria (acute intermittent)**	Uroporphyrinogen I synthetase	Yes
Sandhoff disease	Hexosaminidase A and B	Yes
Tay-Sachs disease	Hexosaminidase A	Yes
Alpha-Thalassemia	Decreased synthesis of alpha-chain hemoglobin	Yes
Beta-Thalassemia	Decreased synthesis of beta-chain hemoglobin	Yes
Wiskott-Aldrich syndrome**	Microthrombocytes	Possible

*- X-linked
**- Autosomal dominant

A pregnant patient with a prior history of an infant with an open neural tube defect carries a 2% recurrence risk and would be a candidate for an amniocentesis. A patient with a first degree family relative delivering an offspring with an open neural tube defect has a 1-2% chance of delivering a similarly affected infant. Pregnant patients in whom there is an open neural tube defect in an indirect family member (nieces, nephews, or cousins) may benefit from a maternal serum AFP determination between the 15th and 20th weeks. Occult spina bifida is not an indication for an amniotic fluid AFP determination.

Before an amniocentesis is performed, usually between 14 and 16 weeks, a discussion of the indications and risks of the procedure is necessary. It is useful for this discussion to be done by an experienced genetic counselor and preliminary information such as blood type, gestational age, and genetic history should be obtained. The risk of fetal loss (1-4%), prematurity, complications of pregnancy or delivery, congenital anomalies or physical injury, or developmental problems of the infant is not increased because of this procedure. Fetal injuries are usually of a minor cutaneous variety. Immediately before the procedure, the patient is again encouraged to ask questions and to be aware that results are not usually available until 1-4 weeks later (depending on the test and laboratory).

Technique

1. An ultrasound examination is routinely performed before, during, and after the amniocentesis to increase the likelihood of a successful initial tap and perhaps lower the risk of fetal loss, premature labor, or delivery complications. By localizing the placenta, the chance of a bloody tap is decreased, thereby minimizing the risk of fetomaternal hemorrhage and a falsely elevated amniotic fluid AFP result. The target site for needle insertion is identified using a plastic straw on the gravid abdomen after the fetal head and thoracic wall have been isolated away from the target site.

2. Local anesthesia may be used but is not usually necessary during the insertion of the 22-gauge spinal needle. Approximately 20 ml of amniotic fluid is withdrawn from the intrauterine sac which is 14-16 weeks size. The total volume of amniotic fluid ranges from 100 ml at 14 weeks, 200 ml at 16 weeks to 300 ml at 18 weeks. The aspiration of meconium-stained fluid occurs infrequently and is not necessarily an ominous sign, but brown fluid (old blood) is associated with an abnormal pregnancy outcome in approximately half the cases. The ultrasound exam should be repeated to look for any malformation of the fetus or gestational sac.

3. When an inadequate specimen is retrieved or the fluid is very bloody, a second needle insertion may be necessary. Ultrasonography with the transducer adjacent to the sterile field is used during the procedure to better localize the needle during insertion. More than two needle insertions should be avoided, and the needles should not be wider than 19-gauge. Although the placenta should be avoided during needle insertion whenever possible, passage of the needle through an anterior placenta has not been associated with an increased risk of complications.

4. A multifetal gestation is discovered in 2% of cases, and each gestational sac may be tapped by inserting the needle under ultrasound guidance. A careful search for two sacs is necessary; however, dyes such as indigo carmine or methyl blue do not need to be instilled.

5. After the needle is withdrawn, an ultrasound examination is performed again, primarily for patient reassurance. The patients are then encouraged to continue their daily routines and expect only mild, transient uterine cramping. Any symptoms of vaginal bleeding, severe cramping, fluid loss, or fever should be reported. Rh-negative, unsensitized patients should receive one vial (300 mg) of Rh immune globulin.

Results

Amniotic fluid is obtained in 94% of the cases with the first needle insertion. Cell culturing is successful in 99% of cases, and the average time from amniocentesis to reporting of karyotype results is 23 days. Alpha-fetoprotein results are usually available in a few days and karyotype results in two weeks. Abnormal karyotypes are found in 1-2% of all cases and communicated directly to the patient's physician instead of to the patient initially. Fetal to maternal bleeding is present in 5-10% of the taps.

Chorionic Villus Sampling: An Alternative

Recent advances in first trimester prenatal diagnosis by chorionic villus sampling (CVS) have increased interest in this procedure which is currently performed primarily at university centers. The CVS has been advantageous in that it may be performed earlier in gestation and the time period from direct preparation of the chorionic villi for cytogenetic results is less. Along with chromosomal studies, other fetal disorders which may be diagnosed by CVS include sickle cell disease, beta thalassemia, and enzymatic diseases. Despite these diagnostic possibilities, the applicability has not been determined for widespread clinical use. Retrieval of chorionic villi and minimizing pregnancy loss are somewhat dependent on the physician experience. Procedure related fetal loss rate appears to be 1%, and other long term complications are minimal.

The procedure is safely performed at 8-13 weeks with the highest success rate at 9-11 weeks. Mild post procedure bleeding is common, but there are generally minimal maternal sequelae. The sampling is performed transcervically using polyethylene tubing with a wire obturator or transabdominally with a 21-gauge spinal needle. The catheter is guided under ultrasound visualization, and villi are aspirated into 5 ml of tissue culture medium in a 20-30 ml syringe. Between two and four aspirations are performed for each patient. The retrieval of tissue has been reliable, and karyotype data have been reported in more than 95% of cases at certain centers. The false negative diagnosis rate is 0.1%; however, there is a 1% frequency of falsely abnormal karyotypes when direct preparations are examined. Therefore, abnormal karyotypes should usually be confirmed from cultured chorionic material and/or subsequent amniotic fluid sampling.

Cervical Cerclage

The most common indication for performing a cervical cerclage is to reinforce an incompetent cervix. An incompetent cervix is defined historically as painless dilation and effacement of the cervix during pregnancy, and its reported incidence varies from 1 in 54 to 1 in 1850 pregnancies. It is identified most commonly during the second trimester (usually 18-26 gestational weeks) and less frequently in the early third trimester. Cervical incompetence should be suspected if premature rupture of membranes or premature labor occurs repeatedly in the second trimester or early third trimester. Women with known in utero DES exposure or in whom an abnormal cervix or uterine cavity have been identified are at increased risk for cervical incompetence. When a 6-8 mm Hegardilator can be easily passed through the internal cervical os in the nonpregnant state, diagnosis of incompetent cervix is suspected. Hysterosalpingography before a subsequent pregnancy may be useful to search for uterine anomalies.

Ultrasound scanning of the lower uterine segment during pregnancy may provide useful information such as: downward protrusion of the amniotic membranes, funneling of the cervix in relation to the upper vagina, thinning of the lower uterine segment, dilatation of the cervical os, or shortening of the cervix. Any such changes on serial ultrasound examinations are suggestive of an incompetent cervix.

Recently, controlled data have been presented which suggest that a prophylactic cervical cerclage may have a beneficial effect in patients with a history of in utero DES exposure, and be useful for the treatment of recurrent hemorrhage from a placenta previa. These indications are controversial.

Technique

1. Before a suture is placed, ultrasound examination is helpful to accurately date the pregnancy, rule out multifetal gestation, localize the placenta, and establish fetal viability.

2. Most cerclage procedures are performed between the 14th and 16th gestational weeks, after any chance for early spontaneous abortion has been excluded and when the risk of infection is lowest. The procedure is usually performed on an outpatient basis.

3. The type of cerclage, McDonald or Shirodkar, is dependent on the individual surgeon's preference as both are equally effective. The McDonald cerclage is used primarily at our institutions, since it is less traumatic and time-consuming and is associated with less blood loss and scarring.

4. Before and after the procedure, fetal heart tones should be sought to rule out the possibility of intrauterine fetal demise.

5. A #2 nylon or #5 mersaline silk suture is used for McDonald cerclages. Whether one or two sutures are placed is dependent on the individual surgeon's preference and the extent of effacement of the cervix. A lead shot may be used when the knot is tied to aid in suture removal later. The suture should be cut several centimeters long to allow easy visability when the McDonald cerclage is removed at or beyond the 37th or 38th week. Mersaline tape is used for the Shiroklar procedure.

6. A subdural (saddle) or epidural regional anesthetic is as acceptable as general anesthesia.

7. If an emergency cerclage is performed with bulging membranes, general anesthesia is administered with the patient in a steep Trendelenburg position. A transabdominal amniocentesis may be necessary to decompress the bulging membranes. The vagina is not cleansed. Several stay sutures using No. 00 silk are attached to the edge of the effaced cervix. The herniated membranes should

fall back in the uterine cavity or may be pushed in using a moist sponge. Two purse-string sutures should then be placed.
8. Antibiotics or sedatives are not required routinely.

Special Considerations

1. Despite the increased risk of premature labor, the finding of a bicornuate or septate uterus or a multifetal gestation alone does not necessitate a cervical cerclage.
2. If there is a history of third trimester premature delivery preceded by premature labor, a cervical cerclage is not routinely necessary. Instead, weekly or biweekly cervical exams are recommended until the third trimester. A cerclage should be promptly placed if there is any dilation of the internal cervical os or if the index finger can be passed into the cervical os. Ultrasound sector scanning of the lower uterine segment may be useful in following these patients.
3. Coital activity may resume in approximately one week after the McDonald procedure. The vaginal incisions for the Shirodkar procedure require 4-6 weeks to heal. The suture and lead shot may cause penile discomfort.
4. Uterine tocolytic drugs such as ritodrine or Delalutin do not need to be given routinely. These should be prescribed only if the patient complains of cramping or if extensive manipulation was required during the procedure.
5. If chorioamnionitis is suspected later, an amniocentesis is helpful to search for any polymicrobial infection.
6. An IUD string retriever is sometimes helpful in retrieving the suture during removal.
7. Transabdominal cervicoisthmic cerclages may be placed if the cervix is too short or if a prior transvaginal cerclage has been unsuccesful.

Mid-Gestation Abortion

Patients desiring pregnancy termination for medical or obstetric indications between 13-24 weeks often go through a process of grief which involves denial, sadness, guilt, anger, and finally acceptance. This is especially true in patients who request abortion for a genetically abnormal or a malformed fetus. These patients are usually older, often married, and desirous of a favorable pregnancy outcome. Furthermore, these patients have usually visualized a living fetus on ultrasound examination before an amniocentesis, and fetal quickening has left an increased feeling of attachment.

Once the decision for pregnancy termination has been made, it should be accomplished without delay, since complications increase with advancing gestational age. Methods available to terminate the pregnancy should be discussed with the patient in an open and honest manner, with advantages and disadvantages being presented in detail. The two methods used for pregnancy termination at our institutions involve prostaglandin vaginal suppositories or surgical dilation and evacuation.

Prostaglandins

Prostaglandin vaginal suppositories are useful for the removal of an intact fetus for morphologic examination and other diagnostic testing to confirm any suspected genetic abnormality or body malformation. Disadvantages to the use of prostaglandin vaginal suppositories include the discomfort of labor, side effects from drug use (nausea, diarrhea, fever), labor, prolonged initiation to delivery interval (mean 14 hrs, range 10-22 hrs), delivery of a liveborn fetus (5%), failure to effect delivery (2-8%), incomplete passage of tissue (10-15%), and retained placenta for two or more hrs requiring operative intervention. Conditions where prostaglandins should be used with caution or are contraindicated are listed in Table 7.3.

Two to four laminaria tents are often wedged within the cervical os 4 hours or more before inserting a suppository to initiate cervical dilation and thereby shorten the initiation-to-abortion time. Because of side effects from the medications, premedication involves an antidiarrheal agent (Lomotil 5 mg orally) and an antiemetic (prochlorperazene) 10 mg IM. Meperidine (50 mg IM and acetaminophen (350 mg rectal suppositories) are often necessary to relieve uterine contraction discomfort and control fevers of 38°C or greater. Administration of further suppositories should be delayed until the maternal temperature is less than 38° C. Otherwise, profound hyperthermia may occur.

Table 7.3
Conditions in which Prostaglandin Therapy Should be Used with Caution or is Contraindicated

Used with Caution	Contraindications
Asthma	Hypersensitivity
Hypertension, hypotension	Active pelvic inflammatory
Cardiovascular disease	disease
Renal disease	Unfavorable fetal position
Peptic ulcer disease	(transverse lie)
Anemia	Placenta previa, complete
Jaundice	
Diabetes mellitus	
Seizure disorder	
Prior uterine surgery	
Fever	

A Prostin 20 mg suppository should be inserted up to the vaginal apex every 3-5 hrs. Careful monitoring of uterine contractions is necessary, and an intrauterine pressure catheter is often helpful. If intense and sustained contractions are noted, a cervical tear or uterine rupture may occur. Persistent sustained contractions may be reversed by removing the suppository and, if necessary, infusion of a beta-adrenergic tocolytic drug. If uterine contractions are inadequate, low doses of oxytocin may also be administered.

Dilation and Evacuation (D & E)

Before 16 weeks gestation, surgical termination is the preferred method, although it may be considered up to 20 weeks in some circumstances. The procedure is rapid and relatively painless, and can be performed on an outpatient basis thereby decreasing medical costs. Disadvantages to dilation and evacuation procedures include the inability to adequately examine the fetus, risks requiring surgical expertise, and potential injury to the cervix or uterine perforation.

Appropriate surgical technique requires sufficient cervical dilation. Three or more medium-size laminaria are usually inserted at least 4 hrs before the procedure. The diameter of cervical dilation should be equal to the number of weeks of gestation plus 2 mm (for example, 18 mm dilation at 16 menstrual weeks). Instruments necessary for sufficient evacuation include Hegar dilators, a non-flexible suction cannula, and strong crushing forceps (example: Sopher forceps).

Most patients prefer to be asleep during the procedure, so general anesthesia is usually administered. Uterine evacuation may also be adequately performed with regional or paracervical anesthesia and sedation. Oxytocin (20 U per liter IV fluid) or methergine(0.2 mg IV slowly) is used routinely during the operation and shortly thereafter to reduce blood loss and risk of infection.

General Precautions

1. Unless uterine evacuation is completed over a short period of time, most patients are prescribed oral ampicillin or tetracycline (such as doxycycline) to reduce postabortion infection rate.
2. The risk of spontaneous abortion or premature labor in subsequent pregnancies is thought to be very low despite the mechanical cervical dilation during these procedures.
3. Rh isoimmunization may result from these pregnancy terminations, since the incidence of sensitization is only slightly less at midgestation than at term. All Rh-negative unsensitized patients should receive a full dose (300 mg) of Rh immune globulin, unless fetal blood obtained during a surgical procedure is found to be Rh-negative.
4. Major abdominal operations such as a hysterectomy or hysterotomy are rarely necessary unless other methods of pregnancy termination are either unavailable or unsuccessful or if a gynecologic complication is present.

Sickle Cell Anemia Transfusion

Sickle cell anemia has been associated in the past with extremely high neonatal and maternal mortality and morbidity rates. To improve the outcome of pregnancies, simple or partial exchange transfusions in gravidas with SS, SC, or S-Thal disease are available. Such transfusions may be undertaken routinely beginning at mid-gestation or the end of the second trimester or may be reserved for complications such as crisis, infection, or symptomatic anemia. Although there are risks associated with partial exchange transfusion, the reported 1% maternal mortality and 20% maternal morbidity rates are usually reduced following exchange transfusion. A cell separator machine allows the patient's plasma, platelets, and leukocytes to be returned with washed compatible donor red cells with Hb AA.

With careful management, a greater than 95% perinatal salvage rate is to be expected with Hb S-S, S-C, and S-Thal. Advantages and disadvantages to partial exchange transfusion are shown in Table 7.4. Close antepartum monitoring of the mother (infection, crisis, thrombosis, worsening anemia, hypertension) and fetus (movement charting, NST, ultrasound) is necessary. Maximum benefit occurs in the first 6-8 weeks following transfusion and declines thereafter because of the shortened lifespan of the stored erythrocytes.

Table 7.4
Value of Partial Prophylactic Exchange Transfusions

Advantages	Disadvantages
Decreased hemoglobin-S concentration	Blood group incompatibility
Increased hemoglobin-A concentration	Allergic reaction
Increased oxygenation	Anaphylaxis
Reduced chance of sickling	Hepatitis, AIDS
Decreased erythropoiesis	Isosensitization
Improved sense of well-being	Febrile reaction
Improved reproductive outcome	Premature labor (?)
Useful in anemia/congestive heart failure	Cost, limited benefits
Decreased maternal infection	Psychologic dependence
Less prolonged hospitalization	
Decreased maternal mortality	

Description of Procedure

1. Notify blood bank personnel well in advance (outpatient transfusion may be considered)
2. Determine hematocrit, hemoglobin-A (Hb-A), and type and cross match the day before anticipated transfusion

3. Initiate IV with lactated Ringer's, to be infused until 200-400 ml given
4. Phlebotomize 500 ml blood into vacutainer (30 min)
5. Give 2 units (150-300 ml/unit) of buffy coat poor, washed red cells (warmed, under pressure over 1-2 hrs)
6. Repeat procedure in afternoon and allow overnight equilibration (total of 4 units of washed erythrocytes)
7. Obtain Hct and Hb-A next morning if inpatient; otherwise, repeat on next clinic visit
8. Discharge patient if Hct over 35 and Hb-A over 40%, respectively, if not, repeat procedure until desired levels obtained
9. Schedule clinic visits every 1-2 weeks with determination of reticulocyte count, Hct, and hemoglobin electrophoresis
10. Repeat entire procedure: 1) at 36-38 weeks, 2) when Hct less than 25% and hemoglobin-A is less than 20%, 3) if crisis occurs, or 4) during labor if necessary.

External Breech Version

Approximately one fourth of fetuses will be in a breech presentation in the early third trimester, but only 3-4% will remain breech at term. Of those pregnancies with a breech fetus at 37 weeks, only 18% will convert to cephalic presentation before delivery. Management of the breech fetus at term involves consideration of the following alternatives: routine cesarean section, selective vaginal delivery, or external cephalic version. External version usually lasts no more than 5 min, and the fetus usually remains in a cephalic position if the version is successful.

Patient Selection

Contraindications for external cephalic version include the following: complications predisposing to uteroplacental insufficiency, twin gestation, fetus with an obvious malformation or suspicious heart rate tracing, fetus that is suspected to be small or large for gestational age, prior uterine surgery, placenta previa or suspected placental abruption.

Although not a contraindication, more difficulties are likely with an obese or primigravid patient.

An inadequate amount of amniotic fluid on ultrasonic exam is also a less favorable prognostic sign. The patient should understand the unlikely but potential risks of the procedure (labor, uterine rupture, cord compression, fetal heart rate abnormality, preterm delivery if performed before 37 weeks) and should be made aware that 35-45% of all attempts will be unsuccessful.

Technique

The procedure should be performed in labor or delivery areas. A reassuring real-time ultrasound examination and a reactive nonstress test should be demonstrated beforehand. Ritodrine to relax the uterus should be infused at a constant rate in low doses. The maternal heart rate, maternal blood pressure, and fetal heart rate should be monitored frequently.

A back flip of the fetus is usually attempted before a forward roll is undertaken. A second examiner should be available to assist in the manipulation, and the procedure should last no more than 5 min. A second attempt after an initial failure may be undertaken only if the mother and fetus remain stable.

The procedure should be discontinued after two or three failed attempts, fetal bradycardia or decelerations, or patient discomfort. If a cesarean section is planned under conduction anesthesia, another attempt at external version may be successful. Fetal heart rate decelerations are uncommon with a successful version. The ritodrine infusion may be stopped after the fetus is turned, but the fetus should be maintained in the new attitude for several minutes. A post-procedure ultrasound exam and a nonstress test should be performed to identify fetal position and any potentially compromised fetus.

Nongenetic Amniocentesis

The most common indication for an amniocentesis during the second half of pregnancy is fetal lung maturity testing. It may also be performed to better evaluate pregnancies complicated by Rh isoimmunization or pelvic infection (usually during premature labor or after preterm ruptured membranes). Ultrasound visualization of the fetal vital parts and the placenta permits selection of a relatively safe pocket of amniotic fluid. After determining that amniocentesis is indicated in select patients the risks of the procedure should be explained, which include: infection, fetal trauma, subplacental hemorrhage, umbilical cord insertion, and fetal death. An operative permit should then be completed. A nonemergent procedure should be scheduled on weekday mornings to ensure that results will be available late that same day.

Technique

The procedure is similar to that described previously for an early gestation genetic amniocentesis. Ultrasound is used before the procedure to determine fetal presentation, fetal BPD, fetal heart activity, placental and umbilical cord localization, and site for needle insertion. Ultrasonography is often used during the procedure to visualize the needle tip. The transducer may be placed near the needle insertion site with a sterile gel or oil being applied on the patient's abdomen. A site away from the placenta, umbilical cord, fetal head, and fetal thorax is ideal. The end of a straw is pressed gently on the skin at the target site.

Aseptic technique is used but a mask, cap, or gown is unnecessary. Local skin anesthesia is recommended for 20-gauge spinal needle with stylet, but a 22-gauge needle may be used without need for local anesthesia. In pregnancies complicated by a multifetal gestation, amniotic fluid should be retrieved from the sac containing an appropriately sized and apparently healthy fetus.

Documentation of the fetal heart rate by auscultation or ultrasound visualization after the procedure is necessary. Nonstress testing is recommended if bloody or meconium-stained amniotic fluid is retrieved. If a nonstress test is already planned, it should be performed after the amniocentesis. The patient should be instructed on fetal movement charting after the procedure. The full (300 mcg) dose of Rh immune globulin should be considered for all Rh-negative unsensitized women (exception: Rh negative fathers) if any blood is retrieved or if the needle is inserted through the placenta.

Suggested Readings

Genetic Amniocentesis and Genetic Counseling

Hook EB: Rates of chromosome abnormalities at different maternal ages. Obstet. Gynecol. 58:282, 1981.

Stephenson SR, Weaver DD: Prenatal diagnosis - A compilation of diagnosed conditions. Am. J. Obstet. Gynecol. 141:319, 1981.

Rodeck CH, Morsman JM: First-trimester chorion biopsy. Br. Med. Bull. 39:338, 1983.

Librach CL, Doran TA, Benzie RJ, et al: Genetic amniocentesis in seventy twin pregnancies. Am. J. Obstet. Gynecol. 148:585, 1984.

Teratology. ACOG Tech. Bull. 84, February, 1985.

Tabor A, Madsen M, Obel EB, et al: Randomised controlled trial of genetic amniocentesis in 4606 low-risk women. Lancet 1:1287, 1986.

Antenatal diagnosis of genetic disorders. ACOG Tech. Bull. 108, September, 1987.

Weiner CP: Cordocentesis for diagnostic indications: Two years' experience. Obstet. Gynecol. 70:664, 1987.

Hanson FW, Zorn EM, Tennant FR, et al: Amniocentesis before 15 weeks' gestation: Outcome, risks, and technical problems. Am. J. Obstet. Gynecol. 156:1524, 1987.

Cervical Cerclage

Olatunbosun OA, Dyck F: Cervical cerclage operation for a dilated cervix. Obstet. Gynecol. 57:166, 1981.

Crombleholme WR, Minkoff HL, Delke I, et al: Cervical cerclage: An aggressive approach to threatened or recurrent pregnancy wastage. Am. J. Obstet. Gynecol. 146:168, 1983.

Harger JH: Cervical cerclage: Patient selection, morbidity, and success rates. Clin. Perinatol. 10:321, 1983.

Lazar P, Gueguen S, Dreyfus J, et al: Multicentred controlled trial of cervical cerclage in women at moderate risk of preterm delivery. Br. J. Obstet. Gynaecol. 91:731, 1984.

Barford DAG, Rosen MG: Cervical incompetence: Diagnosis and outcome. Obstet. Gynecol. 64:159, 1984.

Rush RW, Isaacs S, Mcpherson K, et al: A randomized controlled trial of cervical cerclage in women at high risk of spontaneous preterm delivery. Br. J. Obstet. Gynaecol. 91:724, 1984.

Mid-Gestation Abortion

Harman CR, Fish DG, Tyson JE: Factors influencing morbidity in termination of pregnancy. Am. J. Obstet. Gynecol. 139:333, 1981.

Peterson WF, Berry FN, Grace MR, et al: Second-trimester abortion by dilatation and evacuation: An analysis of 11,747 cases. Obstet. Gynecol. 62:185, 1983.

Mackay HT, Schulz KF, Grimes DA: Safety of local versus general anesthesia for second-trimester dilatation and evacuation abortion. Obstet. Gynecol. 66:661, 1985.

Akhter HH, Flock ML, Rubin GL: Safety of abortion and tubal sterilization performed separately versus concurrently. Am. J. Obstet. Gynecol. 152:619, 1985.

Frank PI, Kay CR, Lewis TLT, et al: Outcome of pregnancy following induced abortion - Report from the joint study of the Royal College of General Practitioners and the Royal College of Obstetricians and Gynaecologists. Br. J. Obstet. Gynaecol. 92:308, 1985.

Methods of midtrimester abortion. ACOG Tech. Bull. 109, October, 1987.

Sickle Cell Anemia Transfusion

Cunningham FG, Pritchard JA, Mason R, et al: Prophylactic transfusions of normal red blood cells during pregnancies complicated by sickle cell hemoglobinopathies. Am. J. Obstet. Gynecol. 135:994, 1979.

Morrison JC, Schneider JM, Whybrew WD, et al: Prophylactic transfusions in pregnant patients with sickle hemoglobinopathies: Benefit versus risk. Obstet. Gynecol. 56:274, 1980.

Nagey DA, Garcia J, Welt SI: Isovolumetric partial exchange transfusion in the management of sickle cell disease in pregnancy. Am. J. Obstet. Gynecol. 141:403, 1981.

Morrison JC, Blake PG, McCoy C, et al: Fetal health assessment in pregnancies complicated by sickle hemoglobinopathies. Obstet. Gynecol. 61:22, 1983.

Nagey DA, Alawode NA, Pupkin MJ, et al: Isovolumetric partial exchange transfusion in the management of sickle cell disease in pregnancy II. Simplified ambulatory technique. Am. J. Obstet. Gynecol. 147:693, 1983.

External Breech Version

Hofmeyr GJ: Effect of external cephalic version in late pregnancy on breech presentation and caesarean section rate: A controlled trial. Br. J. Obstet. Gynaecol. 90:392, 1983.

Phelan JP, Stine LE, Mueller E, et al: Observations of fetal heart rate characteristics related to external cephalic version and tocolysis. Am. J. Obstet. Gynecol. 149:658, 1984.

Ferguson JE, Dyson DC: Intrapartum external cephalic version. Am. J. Obstet. Gynecol. 152:297, 1985.

Hughey MJ: Fetal position during pregnancy. Am. J. Obstet. Gynecol. 153:885, 1985.

Morrison JC, Myatt RE, Martin JN, et al: External cephalic version of the breech presentation under tocolysis. Am. J. Obstet. Gynecol. 154:900, 1986.

Savona-Ventura C: The role of external cephalic version in modern obstetrics. Obstet. Gynecol. Surv. 41:393, 1986.

Ferguson J, Armstrong M, Dyson D: Maternal and fetal factors affecting success of antepartum external cephalic version. Obstet. Gynecol. 70:722, 1987.

Nongenetic Amniocentesis

Garite TJ, Freeman RK, Linzey M, et al: The use of amniocentesis in patients with premature rupture of membranes. Obstet. Gynecol. 54:226, 1977.

Bobitt JR, Hayslip CC, Damato JD: Amniotic fluid infection as determined by transabdominal amniocentesis in patients with intact membranes in premature labor. Am. J. Obstet. Gynecol. 140:947, 1981.

Defoort P, Thiery M: Amniocentesis with the use of continuous real-time echography: Experience with two hundred consecutive cases. Am. J. Obstet. Gynecol. 147:973, 1983.

Jeanty P, Rodesch F, Romero R, et al: How to improve your amniocentesis technique. Obstet. Gynecol. 146:593, 1983.

Bowman JM, Pollock JM: Transplacental fetal hemorrhage after amniocentesis. Obstet. Gynecol. 66:749, 1985.

Savona-Ventura C: Amniocentesis for fetal maturity. Obstet. Gynecol. Surv. 42:717, 1987.

Chapter 8

Intrapartum Monitoring

Induction of Labor

Indications for the induction of labor include documented fetal jeopardy (abnormal fetal heart rate testing), intrauterine growth retardation, premature rupture of membranes more than 12-24 hrs, chorioamnionitis, and removal of a mature fetus from a potentially hostile environment (preeclampsia, poorly controlled diabetes, significant cardiac or pulmonary disorders, neoplasia, postdates). Elective induction for simple convenience is not acceptable.

Successful induction requires both sufficient cervical compliance and adequate uterine contractions. The fact that cervical compliance may be the major factor limiting successful induction has been recognized recently. This has led to the development of several protocols for ripening the unfavorable cervix. Adequate uterine contractions can usually be accomplished through administration of oxytocin.

Initial Assessment

To justify induction, there should be a reasonable assurance of fetal pulmonary maturity, obvious evidence of fetal compromise, or significant threat to the mother's life or long-term health. It is generally believed that the fetus should be in a vertex presentation. While some obstetricians feel induction with a fetus in a breech presentation may be acceptable, most authorities favor cesarean section.

Caution should be employed in the presence of twin gestation, fetal macrosomia, polyhydramnios, a prior low transverse cesarean section, or grand multiparity because of the risk of uterine rupture. Documented fetal/pelvic dysproportion, a previous vertical or classical uterine incision, a previous full-thickness myomectomy, untreated gonorrhea, or active herpes infection are considered absolute contraindications to induction.

The probability of successful induction can be predicted by the Bishop method of cervical scoring (Table 8.1). A Bishop score of 9 or more is almost always associated with successful induction. A score of

Table 8.1
Bishop Score for Assessing the Cervix Before Induction

	0	1	2	3
Dilation (cm)	0	1-2	3-4	5-6
Effacement (%)	0-30	40-50	60-70	80-100
Station	-3	-2	-1, 0	+1, +2
Consistency	Firm	Medium	Soft	
Position	Posterior	Mid	Anterior	

4 or less is consistent with an unfavorable cervix and carries a poor prognosis. Several authorities advocate assigning particular significance to the degree of cervical dilation.

Cervical Priming

The Bishop score (especially cervical dilation) and the probability of a successful induction have been shown to improve using any of the following methods: 1) cervical application of 0.5-3.0 mg of prostaglandin E_2 in a methylcellulose base; 2) stripping of membranes; 3) nipple stimulation or warm soaks to nipples for 1/2 hr three times daily for several days prior to the procedure; or 4) 3-4 intracervical laminaria, usually 12 hrs prior to the procedure.

Prostaglandins are 20-carbon compounds formed by the action of the enzyme, prostaglandin synthetase, which is found in most cells. Prostaglandins released from decidual and myometrial cells are thought to act on specific receptors to alter or inhibit the action of adenyl cyclase, subsequently inhibiting formation of cAMP to eventually bring about changes in smooth muscle tone and modulation of hormonal activity. The intracervical (0.5 mg) or extracervical (2-4 mg) application of a prostaglandin-containing viscous gel has been the subject of much recent interest. Cervices so ripened have led to spontaneous labor, shortened labors, lower cesarean section rates, and more favorable outcomes.

We have prepared the gel by mixing 40 ml of methylcellulose gel with a 20 mg PGE_2 suppository. The final concentration (2 mg/ml) may be stored in a plastic syringe until thawed for use. The cervix is wiped clean prior to gel insertion under direct visualization into the posterior vaginal fornix and cervical os. The patient remains in a supine lithotomy position for at least one hour. Fetal heart rate monitoring should be continuous before and at least one hour after gel insertion. Any subsequent uterine contraction(s) should also be monitored. An infusion of oxytocin may be started as soon as a few hours after gel insertion.

Laminaria may be inserted at any time of gestation, even though their use may not offer a clear advantage during a 2-day induction. Traction using ring forceps on the anterior cervix will allow insertion of at least one medium sized laminaria tent through the internal cervical os. Theoretically, infection in patients treated with laminaria is possible but unlikely. At present it would appear prudent to avoid the use of this method in patients at high risk for infection (ruptured membranes, significant cardiac valve disease).

Oxytocin Administration

Oxytocin is an octapeptide with a half-life of 3-4 minutes and duration of action of approximately 20 minutes. The mechanism by which this agent facilitates smooth muscle contractions is not fully understood, but it is thought to bind to receptors on myometrial cell membranes where cAMP is eventually formed for a dose-dependent increase in amplitude and frequency of uterine contractions. The goal of augmentation or induction of labor is uterine contractions occuring every 2-3 minutes and lasting approximately 45-60 seconds. An intrauterine pressure catheter is often helpful in interpreting uterine activity, and a 50 mm H2O recording is considered to be evidence of an adequate contraction.

An intravenous crystalloid solution should be administered through an 18-gauge intravenous catheter. The oxytocin solution should be piggybacked into this main intravenous line and administered by an accurately calibrated infusion pump. The initial infusion rate of 0.5 mU/min is usually doubled at 15-20 min intervals. The maximum rate of infusion for augmentation is usually no more than 8 mU/min while inductions should generally not exceed 20 mU/min. The uterine response will likely not improve if the rate is 30 mU/min or more. Once sufficient uterine activity has led to adequate progress in labor, the dose of oxytocin should not be increased, rather it should be decreased or stopped to allow labor to continue spontaneously. A hyperstimulatory pattern with contractions overlapping each other may be reversed by discontinuing or decreasing the infusion rate of oxytocin while closely observing the fetal heart rate. If greater than 20 mU/min is required, the dose should be increased by 2 mU every 20 min. This small initial dose, slow rate of incrementation, and need for close monitoring are necessary for the shortest duration from onset of treatment to complete cervical dilation.

Electronic fetal heart rate monitoring is mandatory shortly before and throughout induction or augmentation of labor. Internal monitoring techniques are preferred whenever possible. Three contractions should not occur more frequently than every 10 min and should not last longer than 60-90 sec. If internal monitoring is used, uterine pressures should not exceed 75 mm Hg during a contraction and 30 mm Hg between contractions. Another means of describing uterine activity is using Montivideo units (number of uterine contractions in 10 min multiplied by the mean intensity in mm Hg).

If induction with intact membranes is not successful during the first 12-24 hrs, a repeat attempt is permissible after several hours rest. If a second attempt fails, further attempts are almost never successful. A search for infection is necessary during induction of labor following ruptured membranes for more than 12 hrs.

Intrapartum Fetal Heart Rate Monitoring

Intermittent auscultation and electronic monitoring are the two methods available to monitor the fetal heart rate during labor. Most authorities recommend electronic fetal monitoring in high risk situations which require close intrapartum surveillance. Any additional benefit of electronic fetal monitoring over intermittent auscultation in low risk patients is highly controversial, although nurses and especially physicians often desire electronic monitoring.

Recommendations

1. Both forms of fetal heart rate monitoring during labor (intermittent auscultation and continuous electronic) should be discussed with the patient during the antepartum period and on admission to the labor floor. Her wishes, concerns, and questions about risks, benefits, and limitations should be discussed in an open manner.
2. We recommend and routinely perform a 20 minute tracing on all our patients admitted in early labor. A reassuring tracing coincident with contractions is a favorable prognostic sign of fetal tolerance of labor.
3. Auscultation of the fetal heart rate for 30 sec every 15 min in the active phase of the first stage of labor and every 5 min during the second stage of labor is acceptable for monitoring women at low risk for intrapartum fetal distress. Fetal heart rate changes, particularly bradycardia (less than 120 beats/min), should be sought when the heart rate is auscultated following a uterine contraction.
4. Family centered care and indicated electronic fetal monitoring are not mutually exclusive.
5. Electronic fetal monitoring should never be a substitute for good clinical judgment. The patient's underlying obstetric complication, blood pressure, laboring position, blood loss, and extent of cervical dilation and fetal descent must also be assessed carefully.
6. Conditions which require close intrapartum surveillance and routine electronic fetal monitoring are listed in Table 8.2.
7. In general, direct monitoring by scalp electrode placement provides a more accurate tracing. This technique should be considered when the external tracing is inadequate or suggests fetal compromise. Aseptic and atraumatic technique should be practiced during the placement of the electrode or an intrauterine pressure catheter.
8. The relation between any heart rate abnormalities and uterine contractions should always be sought. When this relation is questioned, an intrauterine pressure catheter should be inserted.
9. Prolonged supine positioning and immobility of the mother should be avoided. The best laboring positions are ambulating or a semi-recumbent, left lateral position.

Table 8.2
Intrapartum Conditions Requiring Electronic Fetal Monitoring

Meconium staining
Use of oxytocin or prostaglandin
Delivery of an anticipated premature, postmature, Rh sensitized,
   growth retarded or macrosomic infant
Medical complications associated with uteroplacental insufficiency
   (hypertension, diabetes, severe anemia, heart disease, renal
   disease)
Presence of abnormal auscultatory findings
Prior cesarean section
Other intrapartum obstetrical complications (failure to progress,
   excessive vaginal bleeding)

---

10. The relation between fetal heart rate decelerations and uterine
    contractions is shown in Figure 8.1.
11. Fetal scalp pH determinations may be useful as an adjunct to
    electronic fetal heart rate monitoring when worrisome fetal heart
    rate patterns are found well before an imminent delivery.

Interpretation

Interpretation of any worrisome fetal heart rate tracing requires
a prior knowledge of the cervical dilation, station, and uterine
contractility. The patient's blood pressure and position and any
medications must be known. Early decelerations (down to 110 beats/min)
are usually associated with normal fetal oxygenation and a normal acid-
base balance. Regardless of the depth, late decelerations are
frequently associated with utero-placental insufficiency and fetal
acidosis. However, the mean time from the start of an abnormal
periodic pattern to the development of fetal acidosis is approximately
1 hr. Therefore, not all infants with late decelerations will be
acidotic when tested in utero nor will they be asphyxiated at birth.
Variable decelerations of the fetal heart rate are common and not
signs of distress unless prolonged, severe, or accompanied by another
heart rate abnormality or an arrest of labor. Severe variable
decelerations (down to 70 beats/min or less with a duration of 60 sec
or more) or a deceleration with a late onset or slow recovery are
frequently associated with fetal hypoxia and acidosis. Variable
decelerations with a late recovery result from a combination of cord
compression and utero-placental insufficiency and have the same
prognosis as late decelerations.
In general, when abnormal heart rate patterns are accompanied by
decreased fetal heart rate variability (0-5 beats/min), the probability
of fetal jeopardy is increased. Late decelerations or
severe variable decelerations are the two most common heart rate
abnormalities related to fetal acidosis. An umbilical cord blood

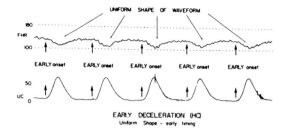

EARLY DECELERATION (HC)
Uniform Shape - early timing

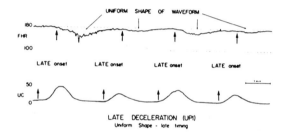

LATE DECELERATION (UPI)
Uniform Shape - late timing

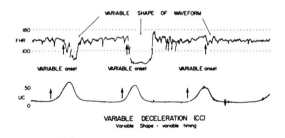

VARIABLE DECELERATION (CC)
Variable Shape - variable timing

Figure 8.1. Fetal heart rate decelerations in relation to uterine contractions. HC - head compression, UPI - uteroplacental insufficiency, CC - cord compression. (From Hon, An Atlas of Fetal Heart Rate Patterns, Harty Press, New Haven, 1968.)

sample for pH and base excess determinations is recommended shortly after delivery under these circumstances.

Fetal heart rate decelerations (especially variables) with a return to the baseline are common during the second stage of labor but are usually mild and of too short a duration to influence fetal outcome. A prolonged deceleration of 90 beats/min or less for 3 min or more or atypical variable decelerations reflect fetal distress and acidosis. This finding is especially true if an abnormal pattern was observed in early labor.

Vaginal Birth after Cesarean

The concept of "once a cesarean section, always a cesarean section" has dominated the practice of American obstetrics for several decades. However, concern over rising cesarean section rates and recognition that a trial of labor with a transverse uterine scar carries a significantly different prognosis from that with a classical scar has led several groups of investigators to reevaluate the need for routine repeat cesarean section. Based on these evaluations, the National Institutes of Health Consensus Committee on Cesarean Section and the American College of Obstetricians and Gynecologists, Committee on Obstetrics: Maternal Fetal Medicine have recommended that a trial of labor is permissible among selected patients with a prior cesarean section.

Antepartum Considerations

1. Uterine rupture occurs in 1-3% of patients attempting vaginal delivery after cesarean section and leads to a perinatal mortality rate of 1/1,000 births. A classical cesarean section is associated with a significantly greater risk of uterine rupture.
2. Approximately two thirds of all patients allowed a trial of labor will deliver vaginally. Those patients who have undergone a prior vaginal delivery or whose prior cesarean section was performed for a nonrecurrent indication have the greatest likelihood (approximately 80%) of delivering vaginally.
3. Recent publications indicate that there is no increased risk of uterine rupture with two prior cesareans. There is very little information regarding outcome in patients with more than two cesareans.
4. Not all patients will deliver vaginally, so any woman undergoing a trial of labor should be aware of the possible need for a cesarean section.
5. The patient should understand that labor pain medication will be used sparingly, particularly during the latent phase of the first stage of labor. The use of regional anesthesia during the active phase of labor has in the past been controversial but is now gaining more widespread acceptance. Refresher childbirth courses are to be encouraged.

6. Patients should understand that a hysterectomy may be necessary if the uterus ruptures, but this is a complication in only approximately 1/1,000 trials of labor.
7. Clinical pelvimetry is essential during the last few weeks before delivery, but x-ray pelvimetry is of little or no value in predicting the likelihood of successful vaginal delivery.

Intrapartum Considerations

1. Two units of whole blood should be typed and screened and an intravenous line should be inserted once labor is established.
2. Oxytocin may be used to augment labor, and close monitoring of uterine contractions (especially using intrauterine catheters) is recommended.
3. Electronic fetal heart rate monitoring is recommended.
4. The anesthesiologists and physician caring for the newborn infant must be notified in advance.
5. There is no evidence to support the prophylactic use of forceps.
6. The same expectations of normal progression during labor (see Figure 9.1) should be applied to patients with a prior cesarean section.
7. Exploration of the uterus after delivery of the placenta is beneficial to assess scar integrity, although its prognostic significance is uncertain.

Delivery at Less Than 25 Weeks

Perinatal mortality rates among very low birth weight infants have dropped dramatically in the last 5 years. Presently, 25 weeks gestation appears to be the break-point at or beyond which a reasonable number of infants can be expected to survive with intensive nursery care. Conversely, aggressive intrapartum management or cesarean section is not justified below this gestational age.

Dating of the pregnancy is extremely important. A falsely low gestational age determination or estimated fetal weight is frequently related to a poorer neonatal outcome. Therefore, it is important to recall that several groups of investigators have reported that ultrasonic parameters of fetal age and growth tend to be smaller among fetuses in premature labor than among fetuses of similar gestational age who ultimately deliver at term. This may lead to underestimation of the true gestational age. The neonatal staff should be notified in advance of any impending delivery. They should also be given the opportunity to talk to the patient along with the staff obstetrician before any management plans are finalized. The patient should be aware that gestational age assessment and the chances of infant survival are accurately determinable only after delivery.

The preferred route of delivery is vaginal, unless gestational dating is questionable or there is any obstruction in the lower genital tract. If dating is uncertain and labor is already established, perinatal survival is not necessarily increased by cesarean delivery.

Uterine activity monitoring is necessary during labor. Fetal heart rate monitoring should not be performed routinely but may be beneficial in changing the mother's position or in giving her oxygen to improve on any heart rate abnormality.

The initial response of any infant weighing 600 gms or more to resuscitative maneuvers is the most important determinant of the infant's chance of survival. A liveborn infant deemed too immature for resuscitation may remain with the parents if they so desire with staff approval. In most cases, such an infant will be brought to the neonatal treatment room for observation in a dignified manner. No live-born infant should be left unattended in the utility room or other undignified location.

In cases of intentional pregnancy termination at a relatively advanced gestational age (such as for progressive hydrocephalus), the attending physician should carefully plan the procedure to ensure fetal demise before delivery or if clinically appropriate, discuss with the patient and her family the possible outcome of a liveborn infant. Physicians should be aware of the statutory definitions and legal requirements governing the reporting of abortions, stillbirths, and immature live births of the state in which they practice. Any liveborn infant will require a birth certificate regardless of length of life.

After delivery of a stillborn fetus or an infant who dies shortly after birth, the obstetric staff should write a note including a detailed description of the fetus as an aid to future counseling and care of the patient. A photograph and body x-ray of the infant are quite often helpful. After delivery, careful inspection of the placenta and the lower genital tract is useful to search for any uterine or placental abnormality. Lastly, a grief response by both parents should be anticipated and supportive care provided.

Magnesium Sulfate

Magnesium sulfate is the most important drug for seizure prophylaxis in patients with severe preeclampsia or eclampsia. In pharmacologic doses, it acts on the central nervous system. Its curariform action at the neuromuscular junction apparently interferes with the release of acetylcholine at motor nerve terminals. Magnesium may also replace calcium at the neuromuscular junction, thereby altering membrane potential and neuromuscular transmission and excitation.

Dosing Regimens

Magnesium sulfate should be given intravenously using a 4-6 gm loading dose over 10-20 min. The usual 2 gm/hr maintenance dose is dependent on the clinical condition of the patient and may be adjusted using an infusion pump.

The patient given magnesium sulfate should be monitored closely for any neuromuscular, respiratory, or cardiac impairment. The following parameters should be monitored carefully: 1) deep tendon reflexes every hour (if absent, the dosage should be lowered), 2) respiratory rate every hour (should be above 12/min), 3) urine output (should exceed 100 ml every 4 hrs, since magnesium is excreted only in the urine).

Serum magnesium levels do not necessarily need to be obtained routinely. However, when the therapy is continued for more than 24 hours, deep tendon reflexes are hypoactive, or anuria is present, a serum magnesium concentration should be drawn. A concentration between 6-8 meq/l is desired. A level between 8-10meq/l is associated with a loss of deep tendon reflexes, while respiratory paralysis develops when concentrations exceed 13-15 meq/l. Cardiac conduction is affected when serum magnesium concentrations exceed 15 meq/l.

An antidote to hypermagnesemia is calcium gluconate or calcium chloride in a 10% solution. A 10 ml (1 gm) dose injected intravenously will usually correct the hypermagnesemia rapidly. Since eclamptic seizures may occur postpartum, intravenous magnesium should be continued for 12-24 hrs along with careful observation of the mother.

Additional Considerations

1. Although magnesium decreases the intrinsic resistance in the uterine vessels, a hypotensive effect does not usually occur or is present only transiently.
2. If a grand mal seizure occurs, magnesium sulfate 4-6 gm intravenously over 20-30 min or diazepam 10 mg intravenously over 2 min should be infused. If the seizure begins despite a maintenance dose of 1-3 gm/hr, a serum magnesium level may be subtherapeutic and 3 gm/hr would be necessary. Concerns about diazepam therapy include its potential respiratory depression and delayed elimination of the principal metabolite.
3. Using seizure prophylaxis doses, magnesium sulfate is thought to have no remarkable effect on impending uterine contractility. Doses used for tocolysis are usually twice those for seizure prophylaxis.
4. The effect of magnesium on the fetus is thought to be minimal, even though serum levels in the fetus rapidly approach those of the mother. Serum magnesium levels in the newborn remain elevated for up to 2 days after delivery. Signs of hypermagnesemia (hypotonicity, lethargy, respiratory depression) occcur most frequently when there has been continuous infusion of magnesium sulfate for more than 24 hrs and when inadequate urinary output is found subsequently in the infant. The neurologic and respiratory performances of the neonate do not necessarily correlate with cord magnesium levels. Neonatal calcium levels are unaffected by intrapartum magnesium therapy.
5. Magnesium therapy should be continued during a cesarean section. A lower dose of a muscle relaxant is usually necessary.

Prophylactic Antibiotics for Cesarean Sections

There has been a 4-fold increase in the incidence of cesarean sections within the past 25 years. Changes in attitudes toward the management of preterm delivery, breech presentation, fetal distress, and midforceps application have influenced those statistics. It is common to expect an increased incidence of postpartum febrile morbidity from infections and prolonged hospitalizations in this group of patients.

At least 30 reports have been published in the English literature within the past decade about the use of broad spectrum prophylactic antibiotics during cesarean section. These drug trials, primarily within the United States, have varied greatly in the choice of antibiotics, treatment schedules, patient populations, and study designs.

Advantages to prophylactic antibiotic therapy include a lowered incidence of febrile morbidity related to endometritis, wound infection, and urinary tract infection when compared with no therapy. Furthermore, patient discomfort, prolonged hospitalization, and patient inactivity are less frequent with antibiotic therapy. Even a short course of a penicillin or cephalosporin antibiotic induces changes within the bacterial flora; however, serious infections caused by anaerobic bacteria are probably not eliminated.

Limitations to prophylactic antibiotic therapy include expense, inability to avoid serious postoperative infections, and questionable value for low-risk surgical patients. Adverse effects from ampicillin or a cephalosporin product are uncommon but may involve hypersensitivity which is reversed with drug discontinuation. Treatment of anaphylactic shock must be undertaken promptly when indicated.

Recommendations

1. Prophylactic therapy must be individualized whenever possible. Infectious control precautions and proper surgical technique with sufficient dilation of the lower uterine segment are essential.
2. An ideal protocol for prophylactic antibiotic therapy has not been established. A single antibiotic with broad spectrum coverage such as ampicillin (500 mg-1 gm) or 1-2 gm of a cephalosporin (i.e. cefazolin, cefoxitin, cephalothin, cefamandole) appears to be as effective as two or more antibiotics combined. No single preparation has been shown clearly to be more effective, and the newer, more expensive antibiotics do not appear to be more beneficial.
3. Certain persons benefit more from perioperative antibiotic therapy, and a review of postoperative infections morbidity by the physician at each hospital is recommended to determine the profile of a patient at moderate or high-risk for developing a pelvic infection. Factors predisposing to endometritis and wound infection include antecedant labor, ruptured amniotic membranes

for 6 hrs or more, multiple vaginal examinations, and lower socioeconomic status.
4. The administration of a drug shortly after cord clamping or surgery is considered to be as effective as administering the drug preoperatively. This protects the unborn infant from antibiotic exposure and avoids masking of neonatal infection.
5. The antibiotic should be administered for less than 24 hrs postoperatively, since cost and potential drug complications are reduced. Febrile morbidity is not significantly greater than if the drug was given 24 hrs or more.
6. Irrigation of the uterus, bladder flap, pelvic cavity, and wound during surgery with a diluted antibiotic solution is an alternative to parenteral therapy. Promising results have been reported with wound and uterine incision irrigation using 2 gms of a cephalosporin such as cefoxitin or cefamandole in 1 liter of normal saline.
7. It is unrealistic to expect every patient to do well postoperatively. Most patients with infectious complications will have endometritis, although other serious pelvic infections must be considered and appropriate cultures obtained before changing the antibiotic therapy. Any antibiotic has the remote possibility of provoking necrotizing enterocolitis.

Suggested Readings

Induction of Labor

Friedman EA, Sachtleben MR, Wallace AK: Infant outcome following labor induction. Am. J. Obstet. Gynecol. 133:718, 1979.

Leake RD, Weitzman RE, Fisher DA: Pharmacokinetics of oxytocin in the human subject. Obstet. Gynecol. 56:701, 1980.

Elliott JP, Flaherty JF: The use of breast stimulation to ripen the cervix in term pregnancies. Am. J. Obstet. Gynecol. 145:553, 1983.

Duff P, Huff RW, Gibbs RS: Management of premature rupture of membranes and unfavorable cervix in term pregnancy. Obstet. Gynecol. 63:697, 1984.

Smith LP, Nagourney BA, McLean FH, et al: Hazards and benefits of elective induction of labor. Am. J. Obstet. Gynecol. 148:579, 1984.

Buchanan D, Macer J, Yonekura ML: Cervical ripening with prostaglandin E_2 Vaginal Suppositories. Obstet. Gynecol. 63:659, 1984.

Macer J, Buchanan D, Yonekura ML: Induction of labor with prostaglandin E_2 vaginal suppositories. Obstet. Gynecol. 63:664, 1984.

Induction of Labor. ACOG Tech. Bull. 110, Nov, 1987.

Intrapartum Fetal Heart Rate Monitoring

Zuspan FP, Quilligan EJ, Iams JD, et al: Predictors of intrapartum fetal distress: The role of electronic fetal monitoring. Am. J. Obstet. Gynecol. 135:287, 1979.

Bowes WA, Gabbe SG, Bowes C: Fetal heart rate monitoring in premature infants weighing 1,500 grams or less. Am. J. Obstet. Gynecol. 137:791, 1980.

Mueller-Heubach E, MacDonald HM, Joret D, et al: Effects of electronic fetal heart rate monitoring on perinatal outcome and obstetric practices. Am. J. Obstet. Gynecol. 137:758, 1980.

Boehm FH, Davidson KK, Barrett JM: The effect of electronic fetal monitoring on the incidence of cesarean section. Am. J. Obstet. Gynecol. 140:295, 1981.

Ingemarsson E, Ingemarsson I, Svenningsen NW: Impact of routine fetal monitoring during labor on fetal outcome with long-term follow-up. Am. J. Obstet. Gynecol. 141:29, 1981.

Wood C, Renou P, Oats J, et al: A controlled trial of fetal heart rate monitoring in a low-risk obstetric population. Am. J. Obstet. Gynecol. 141:527, 1981.

Krebs HB, Petres RE, Dunn LJ: Intrapartum fetal heart rate monitoring V. Fetal heart rate patterns in the second stage of labor. Am. J. Obstet. Gynecol. 140:435, 1981.

Modanlou HD, Freeman RK: Sinusoidal fetal heart rate pattern: Its definition and clinical significance. Am. J. Obstet. Gynecol. 142:1033, 1982.

Greenland S, Olsen J, Rachootin P, et al: Effects of electronic fetal monitoring on rates of early neonatal death, low Apgar score, and cesarean section. Acta Obstet. Gynecol. Scand. 64:75, 1985.

MacDonald D, Grant A, Sheridan-Pereira M, et al: The Dublin randomized controlled trial of intrapartum fetal heart rate monitoring. Am. J. Obstet. Gynecol. 152:524, 1985.

Vintzileos AM, Campbell WA, Dreiss RJ, et al: Intrapartum fetal heart rate monitoring of the extremely premature fetus. Am. J. Obstet. Gynecol. 151:744, 1985.

Leveno KJ, Cunningham FG, Nelson S, et al: A prospective comparison of selective and universal electronic fetal monitoring in 34,995 pregnancies. N. Engl. J. Med. 315:615, 1986.

Ingemarsson I, Arulkumaran S, Ingemarsson E, et al: Admission test: A screening test for fetal distress in labor. Obstet. Gynecol. 68:800, 1986.

Luthy DA, Shy KK, Van Belle G, et al: A randomized trial of electronic fetal monitoring in preterm labor. Obstet. Gynecol. Surv. 42:618, 1987.

Vaginal Birth After Cesarean

Lavin JP, Stephens RJ, Miodovnik M, et al: Vaginal delivery in patients with a prior cesarean section. Obstet. Gynecol. 59:135, 1982.

Gellman E, Goldstein MS, Kaplan S, et al: Vaginal delivery after cesarean section - Experience in private practice. J. Am. Med. Asso. 249:2935, 1983.

Martin JN, Harris BA, Huddleston JF, et al: Vaginal delivery following previous cesarean birth. Am. J. Obstet. Gynecol. 146:255, 1983.

Flamm BL, Dunnett C, Fischermann E, et al: Vaginal delivery following cesarean section: Use of oxytocin augmentation and epidural anesthesia with internal tocodynamic and internal fetal monitoring. Am. J. Obstet. Gynecol. 148:759, 1984.

Finley BE, Gibbs CE: Emergent cesarean delivery in patients undergoing a trial of labor with a transverse lower-segment scar. Am. J. Obstet. Gynecol. 155:936, 1986.

Silver RK, Gibbs RS: Predictors of vaginal delivery in patients with a previous cesarean section who require oxytocin. Am. J. Obstet. Gynecol. 156:57, 1987.

Farmakides G, Duvivier R, Schulman H, et al: Vaginal birth after two or more previous cesarean sections. Am. J. Obstet. Gynecol. 156:565, 1987.

Notzon FC, Placek PJ, Taffel SM: Comparisons of national cesarean-section rates. N. Engl. J. Med. 316:386, 1987.

Delivery at Less Than 25 Weeks

Herschel M, Kennedy JL, Kayne HL, et al: Survival of infants born at 24 to 28 weeks' gestation. Obstet. Gynecol. 60:154, 1982.

Barrett JM, Boehm FH, Vaughn WK: The effect of type of delivery on neonatal outcome in singleton infants of birth weight of 1,000 g or less. J. Am. Med. Asso. 250:625, 1983.

Kariniemi V, Jarvenpa AL, Teramo K: Fetal heart rate patterns and perinatal outcome of very-low-birthweight infants. Br. J. Obstet. Gynaecol. 91:18, 1984.

Socol ML, Dooley SL, Tamura RK, et al: Perinatal outcome following prior delivery in the late second or early third trimester. Obstet. Gynecol. 150:228, 1984.

Kitchen W, Ford GW, Doyle LW, et al: Cesarean section or vaginal delivery at 24 to 28 weeks' gestation: Comparison of survival and neonatal and two-year morbidity. Obstet. Gynecol. 66:149, 1985.

Yu VYH, Loke HL, Bajuk B, et al: Prognosis for infants born at 23 to 28 weeks' gestation. Br. Med. J. 293:1200, 1986.

Amon E, Sibai BM, Anderson GD, et al: Obstetric variables predicting survival of the immature newborn (1000 gm): A five-year experience at a single perinatal center. Am. J. Obstet. Gynecol. 156:1380, 1987.

Magnesium Sulfate

Pritchard JA: The use of the magnesium ion in the management of eclamptogenic toxemias. Surg. Gynecol. Obstet. 100:131, 1955.

Stone SR, Pritchard JA: Effect of maternally administered magnesium sulfate on the neonate. Obstet. Gynecol. 25:574, 1970.

Young BK, Weinstein HM: Effects of magnesium sulfate on toxemic patients in labor. Obstet. Gynecol. 49:681, 1977.

Chesley LC: Parenteral magnesium sulfate and the distribution, plasma levels, and excretion of magnesium. Am. J. Obstet. Gynecol. 133:1, 1979.

Sibai BM, Lipshitz J, Anderson GD, et al: Reassessment of intravenous $MgSO_4$ therapy in preeclampsia-eclampsia. Obstet. Gynecol. 57:199, 1981.

Pritchard JA, Cunningham FG, Pritchard SA: The Parkland Memorial Hospital protocol for treatment of eclampsia: Evaluation of 245 cases. Am. J. Obstet. Gynecol. 148:951, 1984.

Prophylactic Antibiotics for Cesarean Sections

Anstey JT, Sheldon GW, Blythe JG: Infectious morbidity after primary cesarean sections in a private institution. Am. J. Obstet. Gynecol. 136:205, 1980.

Swartz WH, Grolle K: The use of prophylactic antibiotics in cesarean section: A review of the literature. J. Reprod. Med. 26:595, 1981.

Ott, WJ: Primary cesarean section: Factors related to postpartum infection.   Obstet. Gynecol. 57:171, 1981.

Duff P, Gibbs RS, Jorgensen JH, et al: The pharmacokinetics of prophylactic antibiotics administered by intraoperative irrigation at the time of cesarean section.   Obstet. Gynecol. 60:409, 1982.

Rudd EG, Cobey EA, Long WH, et al: Prevention of endomyometritis using antibiotic irrigation during cesarean section.   Obstet. Gynecol. 60:413, 1982.

Ford LC, Hammil HA, Lebherz TB: Cost-effective use of antibiotic prophylaxis for cesarean section.   Am. J. Obstet. Gynecol. 157:506, 1987.

Duff P: Prophylactic antibiotics for cesarean delivery: A simple cost-effective strategy for prevention of postoperative morbidity.   Obstet. Gynecol. 157:794, 1987.

Chapter 9

Intrapartum Complications

Abnormal Labor

An evaluation for progress during labor should be based on a comparison with carefully established normal ranges. The strength of the uterine contractions depends on their frequency and duration and the indentability of the uterus. Adequate contractions leading to progressive cervical dilation usually occur every 2-3 minutes and last 45-60 seconds, and the firm uterus is not indentable.

We routinely chart the cervical dilation and station as a function of time. The first stage of labor occurs from the onset of true labor to complete cervical dilation and typically lasts 6-18 hours in nulliparous and 2-10 hours in multiparous women. The second stage from complete dilation of the cervix until birth usually lasts 30 minutes to 3 hours in nulliparous and 5-30 minutes in multiparous women.

Protracted or arrested cervical dilation occurs during the early (latent) and late (active) phases of the first stage and during the second stage (Figure 9.1). Caput formation of the fetal scalp, a failure of proper fetal descent into the pelvis, fetal macrosomia, and a poor fetal heart rate response to stressful uterine contractions are often present. Intervention before prolonged abnormal labor should minimize fetal compromise and reduce the incidence of neonatal morbidity.

Proposed Management

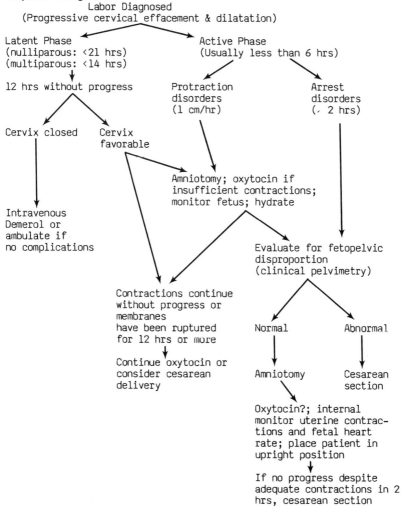

Labor Diagnosed
(Progressive cervical effacement & dilatation)

Latent Phase
(nulliparous: <21 hrs)
(multiparous: <14 hrs)

Active Phase
(Usually less than 6 hrs)

12 hrs without progress

Protraction
disorders
(1 cm/hr)

Arrest
disorders
(< 2 hrs)

Cervix closed

Cervix
favorable

Intravenous
Demerol or
ambulate if
no complications

Amniotomy; oxytocin if
insufficient contractions;
monitor fetus; hydrate

Evaluate for fetopelvic
disproportion
(clinical pelvimetry)

Contractions continue
without progress or
membranes
have been ruptured
for 12 hrs or more

Continue oxytocin or
consider cesarean
delivery

Normal

Abnormal

Amniotomy

Cesarean
section

Oxytocin?; internal
monitor uterine contrac-
tions and fetal heart
rate; place patient in
upright position

If no progress despite
adequate contractions in 2
hrs, cesarean section

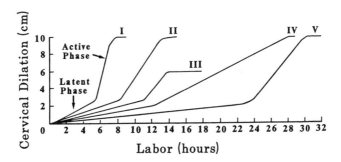

Figure 9.1. Phases of normal and abnormal cervical dilation during the first stage of labor. (I - average multipara, II - average primigravida, III - arrested active phase, IV - prolonged active phase, V - prolonged latent phase).

Meconium

The passage of meconium-stained amniotic fluid during labor occurs in 20-25% of all vaginal deliveries and may indicate fetal distress. Although there may be no apparent sign of fetal distress, it may be a consequence of hypoxia or anoxia leading to a relaxation of the fetal anal sphincter and rectum with increased bowel peristalsis and intrauterine gasping. Unlike term and postterm fetuses, the premature fetus infrequently or rarely passes meconium and has an extraordinary capacity to withstand signs of severe distress for many hours until intrapartum death.

Other conditions in which meconium is observed include breech presentation, cord entanglements, prolonged labor, toxemia of pregnancy, and postdate pregnancies. These neonates require resuscitation, respiratory support, and antibiotics more frequently than the general newborn population.

Recommendations

1. Expedient or operative delivery is not indicated because of meconium staining alone. A search for any antepartum or intrapartum complication(s) is necessary.

2   The passage of meconium in breech presentations is caused by pressure of uterine contractions on the fetal intestines and is not necessarily a sign of fetal distress.
3. When meconium is passed at any time during labor, electronic fetal heart rate monitoring is necessary. Thick or early heavy meconium is especially associated with asphyxia and acidosis.
4. Should there be a significant alteration in the fetal heart rate, immediate delivery may be needed to save the infant.
5. A DeLee suction trap should be used to vigorously suction the infant's oropharynx, nasopharynx, and gastric aspirate before delivery of the infant's shoulder. In the event that labor is too rapid for maternal transport to the delivery room, a DeLee suction trap should be located in each laboring room.
6. After delivery, the newborn's vocal cords should be visualized, and the trachea intubated and suctioned.
7. Not all green amniotic fluid is meconium. This may instead represent vomited bile secondary to a gastrointestinal obstruction.

Fetal Scalp pH Sampling

Respiratory and metabolic acidosis is apt to occur in the fetus when episodes of repetitive severe variable or late decelerations or prolonged bradycardia of the fetal heart rate are observed, with or without a loss of beat-to-beat variability. When a worrisome tracing is present, the clinician should reassess any underlying complication, search for excess vaginal bleeding, determine the mother's blood pressure, and perform a bimanual examination (cervical effacement and dilation, extent of fetal descent, rule out a prolapsed cord).

If the tracing remains worrisome despite oxygen therapy and a change in maternal position, the following steps should be taken: 1) recheck the cervix, 2) discontinue any oxytocin, 3) attempt to correct any underlying complication, and 4) assess the acid-base status of the fetus by scalp pH sampling.

Fetal blood sampling is performed in approximately 3% of our laboring patients. It is not usually performed until the cervix is 3 cm dilated or more. Careful technique is necessary, especially if the fetus is premature. The technique is to be avoided in mothers known to be carriers of hemophilia, other bleeding disorders, or genital infections such as herpes.

Technique

1. The patient should be in a dorsal lithotomy position with a left lateral tilt.
2. The vaginal vault should be cleaned with a Betadine solution.
3. The endoscope with a connected light source is inserted into the vagina against the presenting fetal part.
4. The puncture area is cleaned with a swab, and silicone gel is applied.

5. A 2 mm deep skin puncture is performed using a special guarded lancet so that an adequate amount of free-flowing blood will pass into the heparinized capillary tube.
6. A metal flea is inserted into the blood-filled capillary tube and maneuvered using a magnet.
7. The tube is sealed, placed on ice, and promptly sent to be analyzed.
8. Hemostasis of the puncture site is accomplished by direct pressure for at least one full uterine contraction.
9. Attention should be placed on any acceleration of the fetal heart rate. Such a finding is reassuring after either pinching of the scalp with a clamp or insertion of a lancet.

Interpretation

An acceleration of the fetal heart rate is expected after the blood sampling when the pH is more than 7.25. In contrast, no acceleration is expected after scalp puncture when the pH is 7.20 or less. A scalp pH of 7.20 or less is strongly suggestive of fetal asphyxia and acidosis. If 7.20-7.25, another scalp pH should be determined in 15-30 min especially if there is an abnormal tracing or a less than rapid progression in labor. A pH of more than 7.25 is considered to be normal but should be repeated in 1 hr or less if the abnormal heart rate pattern persists or worsens.

Complications

Infection is unlikely in properly selected patients sampled using aseptic technique. Bleeding should be controlled with pressure, and a skin clip is rarely necessary.
A broken blade is a rare event, but inspection of the blade is necessary after puncture. A magnet near the incision site will be helpful in withdrawing any blade. X-ray localization may be necessary.
The greatest benefit with scalp pH determinations is the ability to delay or avoid a cesarean section in the presence of a reassuring pH result. A persistently worrisome heart rate tracing should be acted upon without delay before acidosis becomes evident.

Breech Delivery

The overall incidence of breech presentation at term is approximately 3%. The incidence is substantially higher at earlier gestational ages, being 40% at less than 28 weeks and 17% between 28-31 weeks. Breech presenting fetuses are at increased risk of perinatal mortality and morbidity from not only birth trauma but also because the presentation is associated with conditions or complications such as prematurity, low birth weight for gestational age, prolapsed cord, congenital malformations, placenta previa and abruptio placenta.
Many vaginal deliveries occur when the mother presents in late labor and the cervix is nearly completely dilated. In cases wherein

there is sufficient time for a decision, most authorities believe that carefully selected breech fetuses can safely deliver vaginally, and house officers are provided the opportunity to acquire skills in vaginal breech delivery. Hazards to breech delivery must be recognized, and cesarean section is the route of delivery in at least three fourths of circumstances in our experience.

Route of Delivery

Cesarean Section
An understanding of indications for cesarean section must be understood. These are listed in Table 9.1. An ultrasound examination to localize the placenta, rule out twins, and search for a fetal anomaly is useful before surgery.
A low transverse uterine incision is satisfactory if there is adequate room to avoid unnecessary trauma to the aftercoming fetal head. This incision is associated with decreased postoperative morbidity and will permit a trial of labor and attempt at vaginal delivery with any subsequent pregnancies. If the lower uterine segment is not well developed, as is often seen in premature or low birth weight breech fetuses, a vertical uterine incision may be preferable to minimize entrapment of the fetal head.

Vaginal Delivery
Prerequisites for a trial of labor include the following findings: 1) no other indications for cesarean section, 2) frank breech presentation, 3) EFW 2,500 to 3,800 gm by two examiners, 4) gestational age 36 weeks or more, 5) no space-occcupying malformation or twins, 6) adequate medical personnel (another obstetrician, anesthesiologist/anesthetist, pediatrician), and 7) normal clinical or x-ray pelvimetry. Approximately half of these candidates will have

Table 9.1
Indications for Cesarean Delivery of the Breech Fetus

Footling and complete breech presentations with EFW $>$ 750 gm, or gestational age 26 weeks or more
Frank breech presentations with EFW less than 2,500 gm or more than 3,800 gm, or gestational age less than 36 weeks
Hyperextension of fetal head
Insulin-dependent diabetes mellitus
Floating presenting part
Pelvic contracture by x-ray or clinical pelvimetry
History of prior difficult or traumatic delivery or perinatal death
Any coexistent obstetric indication for cesarean section whether or not they receive oxytocin

---

inadequate pelvic measurements on x-ray examination. Once all prerequisites are met, approximately half will safely deliver vaginally.
Anesthesia and neonatal personnel should be notified in advance. The patient's blood should be typed and screened. Internal fetal heart rate and uterine activity monitoring is essential. Progressive cervical dilation (1.5 cm/hr) and sufficient descent of the presenting part during the active phase of labor must occur. Oxytocin may be used judiciously to augment uterine contractions to reach a 50 mm Hg intensity at a rate of 3 per 10 minute period.
Compared with a total extraction, a controlled or partial breech extraction minimizes trauma. A well-controlled and properly-executed breech extraction is safer for both mother and fetus than a hastily-performed, difficult cesarean section. A second physician is necessary to assist in the extraction process. During any cesarean delivery after a trial of labor, another person may be necessary to push up the presenting part out of the maternal pelvis.

Midforceps Delivery or Vacuum Extraction

An arrest of fetal descent at the mid-pelvis is a common intrapartum complication. Accurate determination of the depth of fetal head descent into the pelvis is essential before midforceps or vacuum application is attempted. A cesarean section is necessary when a floating fetal head persists despite an adequate trial of labor. Once the widest diameter of the presenting part has passed through the inlet (engagement), an abdominal operation with an assistant pushing the presenting part upward may not be necessary if forceps can be applied and used properly. If fetal distress occurs suddenly, an attempt at midforceps or vacuum delivery may be undertaken with caution.

Midforceps Application

Before application of the forceps, a staff physician should reassess the fetal position. Manual rotation should be attempted beforehand, since forceps delivery may be quite difficult if no rotation can be performed manually. The pediatricians should be notified in advance before application of the forceps, and close monitoring of the fetal heart rate is necessary in the delivery room.
Forceps should be applied only after the cervix is completely dilated and there is no evidence of cephalopelvic disproportion. Forceps may be applied only after the biparietal diameter has passed through the inlet, and the skull has reached the ischial spines (station 0-2+). A senior house officer or faculty member should check the forceps application before any rotation is undertaken. Traction on the fetal head should be along the least resistant pathway of the pelvis. Excess force should be avoided, especially in any incorrect line of access into the pelvis.
After delivery, the genital tract and infant should be examined carefully. Lacerations of the supporting pelvic tissues, tears of the

cervix or uterus, or injury to the bladder and rectum should be sought. Injury to the fetus should also be sought and documented. These injuries include an intracranial hemorrhage (subdural, epidural, subarachnoid), linear or depressed skull fracture, brachial plexus injury, cephalohematoma formation, facial paralysis, clavicular fracture, and bruising.

Vacuum Extraction

The vacuum extractor is another instrument used to assist the mother's efforts to expel the term, vertex fetus. The principal extractors which are available consist of soft rubber rather than metal cups. Two vacuum extractors commonly used are the silastic cup and the smaller MityVac vacuum delivery system. Advantages of the vaccuum extractor include less force being applied to the fetal vertex, reduced anesthesia requirements, ease of application, and ease for the head to find its path out of the maternal pelvis. Disadvantages of the extractor include traction applied only during contractions, use limited to term infants, prolonged delivery when compared to forceps, and care to maintain the vacuum. Morbidity and mortality are low, but caput formation for several hours is quite common.

The vacuum extractor is to be applied to term infants with a vertex presentation after the cervix has become fully dilated and effaced. The head must be engaged with the membranes being ruptured. No vaginal mucosa or cervical tissue should be caught between the vacuum and fetal head. Vacuum pressures can be increased almost instantaneously. A vacuum pressure of up to 50 cm Hg should be obtained and maintained during traction. When maintaining this pressure, it is easier for the cup to conform to the fetal head and allow proper traction.

Traction should be applied during a contraction with the mother bearing down. Traction should be in a plane perpendicular to that of the cup application, since improper traction may cause scalp laceration or subglial hemorrhage. A safety feature of the vacuum cup is its inability to remain on the fetal head during excess traction. The vacuum pressure should be minimal between contractions. The operator's hand should be maintained on the cup, so that if the cup disengages inadvertently, it will not move freely through the vaginal canal and trap maternal tissue. Although both types of cups seem adequate, the MityVac cup seems to hold more suction as the head is delivered, with less need for application of outlet forceps.

Prolapse of the Umbilical Cord

A prolapse of the umbilical cord occurs in 0.3-0.6% of all pregnancies. It is an obstetric emergency which is commonly associated with a breech presentation, polyhydramnios, premature delivery, early artificial rupture of the amniotic membranes, and malpresentation of the fetus. Perinatal mortality can be as high as 35% without immediate temporary therapy and prompt delivery.

A prolapsed umbilical cord may be ignored when the fetus is either already dead, has a major malformation incompatible with life, or is so immature that survival is improbable.

Temporary Therapy

The examiner's hand should be placed in the vagina to ascertain the cervical dilation, station, and presenting part. The presenting part should be pushed up and away from the umbilical cord as the patient is placed in a knee-chest or Trendelenburg position.

The mother should be given oxygen by mask, and the fetal heart rate should be monitored continuously by auscultation or ultrasound imaging. Further assistance by a senior house officer or faculty member is necessary, and the anesthesia and neonatal staff should be notified promptly. Inserting a Foley catheter to distend the bladder and administering a beta agonist (ritodrine 350 mcg or terbutaline 250 mcg) intravenously over 5 minutes may alleviate cord compression.

Delivery Considerations

Cervical dilation is perhaps the most important prognostic indicator. A cervix which is inadequately dilated and a delay of over 30 min increases fetal mortality significantly. Cesarean section is the best method of delivery, unless the cervix is dilated completely and the fetal head is low in the pelvis. Under this circumstance, fundal pressure and forceps should be applied to expedite vaginal delivery. If the cervix is incompletely dilated, manual dilation of the cervix is necessary as the cord is repositioned to avoid further compression.

In addition to fetal heart rate monitoring, the cord should be palpated for any pulsation while the mother is in the Trendelenburg position. Ultrasound visualization is also helpful especially when the fetal heart rate is difficult to locate. The neonatal staff should be in attendance to institute immediate resuscitation of the newborn.

Postoperative febrile morbidity and signs of infection become evident invariably. Parenteral antimicrobial therapy during the immediate postoperative period is recommended using broad-spectrum antibiotics (cefoxitin, penicillin and gentamicin, penicillin and clindamycin, clindamycin and gentamicin).

Emergency Cesarean Section

Between 20-25% of gravidas are now delivered by cesarean section. Approximately two-thirds of these procedures are performed after the onset of labor and are more likely to be considered emergency cesarean sections. It may be appropriate to subdivide this group into those requiring truly emergent surgery (intrapartum fetal distress, prolapsed cord, ruptured uterus, severe abruptio placenta, placenta previa with extensive hemorrhage) or urgent surgery (cephalopelvic disproportion, abnormal presentation, worrisome antepartum fetal heart testing, placenta previa with mild bleeding). Immediate delivery is required in the former category, whereas reasonably rapid intervention is required in the latter. It is important for the obstetric service at every hospital to have well-defined protocols for the performance of emergent and urgent cesarean sections.

Maternal Preparation

Blood samples should be sent routinely for a complete blood count and type and screen. A platelet count, prothrombin time, partial thromboplastin time, fibrinogen, and fibrin split products should be determined in patients with excessive uterine bleeding.

Pulmonary aspiration of gastric contents remains the leading cause of anesthetic maternal mortality. Every gravida should receive oral antacid prophylaxis (such as sodium citrate) every 3 hrs during labor. This therapy raises the pH of gastric contents (usually from 2.5 to 4) to decrease the severity of any aspiration during induction of general anesthesia. Various pharmacologic approaches to decrease acidity (such as cimetidine) and reduce the volume of gastric contents (such as metoclopramide) are being studied.

The abdomen should be shaved and a Foley catheter inserted when the potential need for an emergency or urgent cesarean section is recognized. It may be prudent to move the patient and allow her to labor in the delivery room. Fetal monitoring should be continued while in the delivery room.

Significant maternal metabolic disorders, hypoxia, and hypovolemia should be corrected. Maternal cardiopulmonary and neurologic function should be stable before induction of anesthesia.

Medical Personnel Preparation

Provisions for performing a cesarean section within 15 min would be available at any tertiary obstetrical service, and to achieve this adequate personnel must be available on an around-the-clock basis. Each member of the surgical, anesthesia, and nursing team must understand his or her responsibility in preparing for cesarean delivery. In less well-staffed hospitals, appropriate personnel should be notified when a potential problem is first recognized as opposed to when the actual decision is made to perform a cesarean section. Although there may be false alarms, this practice avoids an unnecessary and potentially disastrous delay.

Primary and back-up scrub and circulating nurses should be clearly identified on each nursing shift. Anesthesia personnel responsible for cesarean sections should be notified of problems in advance if possible. Neonatal personnel should also be notified of potential problems for they may also wish to interview the patient and evaluate her problem in the obstetrician's presence.

Technique

A rapid sequence induction with general anesthesia and endotracheal intubation is the preferred technique for most emergency cesarean sections. Although some highly experienced obstetric anesthesiologists prefer to inject an epidural catheter if it is already in place, preparation for administering general anesthesia is necessary if the epidural does not provide rapid anesthesia. There is usually sufficient time to administer a regional anesthetic in the case of an urgent cesarean section. While maximum surgical speed is necessary in emergency situations, maternal safety should never be sacrificed to haste.

A Betadine spray to the abdomen and insertion of a Foley catheter are usually adequate for a truly emergent cesarean section. Operative delivery using local anesthesia is not considered to be faster than waiting for general anesthesia administration.

A vertical abdominal incision provides more rapid access to the uterus during emergency situations. There is usually no need to clamp minor bleeders or ligate major bleeders before delivery of the infant. Once the uterine incision has been made with a scalpel, it can be extended rapidly by stretching with the surgeon's fingers. A bladder injury should be sought and if present, repaired with two layers of interrupted 3-0 chromic suture in an imbricating manner. Methylene blue or sterile formula may be injected above the clamped Foley catheter to determine the extent of any tear and to see if the repair is adequate.

There should be sufficient nursing personnel available to assist the anesthesiologist, anesthetist, or pediatrician with infant resuscitation as well as to assist the surgeons and anesthesiologists with care of the mother.

Shoulder Dystocia

True shoulder dystocia is uncommon but represents a very stressful intrapartum condition requiring vaginal delivery. It may be anticipated beforehand under the following circumstances: prolonged second stage of labor, fetal macrosomia, anencephaly, locked twins, enlargement of the fetal abdomen or thorax, and maternal diabetes.

Method of Delivery

A senior house officer or staff member and anesthesiologist should be notified at once for further assistance. The mother's hips should be more fully flexed in the direction of her chest. An inhalational anesthetic such as halothane should be administered by an anesthesia staff member for complete muscle relaxation. An episiotomy, preferably large, should be made. In some instances a second episiotomy may be helpful.

Gentle upward traction on the delivered head should be performed as the patient is told to bear down or as pressure on the fundus is applied by an assistant. If this fails on one or two efforts, an attempt should be made to either deliver the anterior shoulder, extract the posterior shoulder or arm, or "corkscrew" the shoulders using the Wood's maneuver.

Delivery of Anterior Shoulder

The examiner's hand is placed behind the anterior shoulder, and the shoulder is rotated into the oblique diameter of the pelvis with the next uterine contraction. Suprapubic pressure is exerted. Firm, downward traction on the head is necessary to bring the anterior shoulder in and out of the pelvis. The obstetrician's forefinger may also be hooked under the axilla as early as possible during the extraction procedure.

Extraction of Posterior Shoulder and Arm

The examiner's hand may instead be placed behind the posterior shoulder with the arm being grasped and carried over the front of the infant's abdomen. Once the hand is seized, it can be extracted with the arm to permit the anterior shoulder to be either delivered under the pubic arc or rotated 180° and delivered in the posterior position.

Corkscrew Rotation

Instead of grasping the posterior arm and delivering the hand, the front of the posterior shoulder is pressed so that the shoulder moves with force with the back leading the way. It is rotated 180 until the posterior shoulder is delivered under the pubic arc. After delivering the posterior shoulder, the anterior shoulder is now posterior. Continued downward pressure on the fetus' buttocks by fundal pressure should permit another rotation of 180° in the same direction so that the shoulder is delivered under the pubic arc.

Preparation for the Compromised Infant

The quality of intrapartum care, resuscitation, and immediate neonatal care often determines whether a compromised infant will survive or suffer from extensive morbidity. Careful preparation is required before delivery. When a recognized antepartum complication is present, the pediatrician should be notified before the induction of labor or performance of a cesarean section.

Intrapartum

Unless there has been a prior antepartum complication, a compromised fetus is usually not anticipated until after the onset of labor. The presence of a fetal malpresentation, meconium staining, failure of descent, or abnormal heart rate pattern suggests fetal compromise. Under any of these circumstances, the pediatricians should be notified in advance.

The observation of a worrisome heart rate pattern (bradycardia, loss of beat-to-beat variability, or repetitive late or severe variable decelerations) warrants continuous electronic monitoring, frequent pelvic examination, reassessment of any underlying complication, and fetal scalp pH determination. Trauma to the fetus should be minimized, and oxygen should be given to the mother before and during any difficult deliveries.

Excessive maternal sedation and prolonged inhalational anesthesia should be avoided; instead, local or conduction anesthesia is preferred. After delivery, cord blood should be sampled and sent for pH and base excess determinations. We collect blood from the umbilical vein in a syringe and place it in a heparinized vacutainer. A pH value of less than 2.5 and base excess lower than -7 reflect respiratory acidosis. Apgar scores should also be assigned at 1 and 5 min after delivery using the scoring system shown in Table 9.2.

Table 9.2
Apgar Scoring System

	0	1	2
Heart rate	Absent	Below 100 bpm	Over 100 bpm
Respiratory effort	Absent	Slow, irregular	Good crying
Muscle tone	Flacid	Some flexion of extremities	Active motion; flexed extrem.
Reflex irritability	No response	Grimace	Vigorous cry
Color	Blue; pale	Body pink; extremities blue	Completely pink

Newborn Care

After delivery, a potentially compromised infant should be handled gently, dried immediately, and kept warm in an area with properly controlled temperature and humidity. The upper airway should be cleared, and the head should be positioned down at an angle of 30° with the horizontal. The upper airways should be suctioned of any mucous and debris.

Oxygen is the best drug therapy until the infant's respiratory center can maintain its regulatory function. Oxygen administered using a well-fitting mask may act as a physiologic stimulant to the anoxic respiratory center along with maintaining pulmonary ventilation. Direct endotracheal intubation with positive pressure ventilation is necessary when respiratory difficulties are encountered despite these initial measures.

Narcotic-induced depression of the newborn is uncommon, and proper resuscitation and adequate supportive care should diminish any need for a narcotic antagonist. Naloxone (Narcan), an almost pure opioid antagonist with minimal agonist action, is the drug of choice for narcotic induced depression. The neonatal preparation (0.02 mg/ml) is recommended at a dose of 0.1 mg/kg IV. Less predictable absorption occurs with subcutaneous, intramuscular and intralingual administration. To ensure lasting action, naloxone may be readministered within 5 minutes of an initial positive response if rhythmic respirations are not sustained. Routine use of this narcotic antagonist would not seem appropriate after delivery, and the long term safety of naloxone is uncertain.

Established protocols for treatment of newborn brain edema, hypoperfusion, hypoxia, acidosis, and hypoglycemia are necessary. After resuscitation, it is necessary to monitor the infant closely for any signs of hypotonicity, irritability, jitteriness, seizures, or feeding problems. Potentially correctable metabolic disorders would include hypoglycemia, hyperbilirubinemia, and calcium imbalance.

Along with close observation, antibiotics are often indicated when sepsis is suspected. These drugs are begun after appropriate cultures have been obtained. Signs of systemic hypotension in the neonate should be sought and corrected as quickly as possible. Since severe fetal-maternal hemorrhage may explain birth asphyxia or death in an anemic infant, a Kleihauer-Betke test of the mother's blood should be determined.

Subsequent Development

All stages of fetal and neonatal development influence normal neurologic outcome. Most neurologic disorders are not directly linked to a specific prenatal and perinatal event, and it cannot be said with any degree of certainty that mental retardation, cerebral palsy, and epilepsy are due to mild asphyxia. Physician attitude is very important, however, since a given fetus assessed to be viable (at least 25 weeks or 600 grams) is more likely to survive with immediate attention. Improved obstetric techniques have reduced the number of cases of brain disease resulting from birth trauma from prolonged or difficult labor, difficult forceps delivery, or obstetric trauma. The nature, frequency, and severity of brain disorders are affected by such factors as race, socioeconomic status, lifestyle, and environmental influences both before and after birth. Social interaction of the infant and child with family, school acquaintances, and peers may play a role in the severity of their affliction.

Pure mental retardation or grand mal seizures are rarely associated with intrapartum events. Birth trauma and asphyxia (the inability to breathe associated with the reduced oxygen supply to the brain) singly or together are infrequent causes of mental retardation, although they can cause brain disorders. Less than 15% of cases of severe mental retardation (IQ less than 50) can be attributed to perinatal events. Prenatal genetic counseling, diagnosis of chromosomal defects, and rapid intervention with neonates who have metabolic disorders can reduce the incidence and severity of the retardation. Social, economic, and cultural factors associated with prematurity and intrauterine growth retardation are related to mild mental retardation. Future prenatal counseling should include topics such as proper nutrition, avoidance of smoking, drugs, and alcohol abuse, and continuation of maternal education.

Although specific events within the intrapartum period may explain a significant portion of cerebral palsy, the illness is often linked with compounding factors such as low birth weight and asphyxia. Severe asphyxia and prematurity are the only two major identifiable causes of cerebral palsy, but almost three-quarters of children with cerebral palsy have no evidence of such asphyxia. Furthermore, three-quarters of severely asphyxiated infants who survive demonstrate no major handicap by the time they reach school age. In the presence of neonatal seizures, there is a high risk of the later development of cerebral palsy and epilepsy.

Suggested Readings

Meconium

Meis PJ, Hall M, Marshall JR, et al: Meconium passage: A new classification for risk assessment during labor. Am. J. Obstet. Gynecol. 131:509, 1978.

Starks GC: Correlation of meconium-stained amniotic fluid, early intrapartum fetal pH, and Apgar scores as predictors of perinatal outcome. Obstet. Gynecol. 56:604, 1980.

Krebs HB, Petres RE, Dunn LJ, et al: Intrapartum fetal heart rate monitoring III. Association of meconium with abnormal fetal heart rate patterns. Am. J. Obstet. Gynecol. 137:936, 1980.

Meis PJ, Hobel CJ, Ureda JR: Late meconium passage in labor - A sign of fetal distress? Obstet. Gynecol. 59:332, 1982.

Dooley SL, Pesavento DJ, Depp R, et al: Meconium below the vocal cords at delivery: Correlation with intrapartum events. Am. J. Obstet. Gynecol. 153:767, 1985.

Davis RO, Philips JB, Harris BA, et al: Fetal meconium aspiration syndrome occurring despite airway management considered appropriate. Am. J. Obstet. Gynecol. 151:731, 1985.

Fetal Scalp pH Sampling

Zanini B, Paul RH, Huey JR: Intrapartum fetal heart rate: Correlation with scalp pH in the preterm fetus. Am. J. Obstet. Gynecol. 136:43, 1980.

Young DC, Gray JH, Luther ER, et al: Fetal scalp blood pH sampling: Its value in an active obstetric unit. Am. J. Obstet. Gynecol. 136:276, 1980.

Clark SL, Gimovsky ML, Miller FC: The scalp stimulation test: A clinical alternative to fetal scalp blood sampling. Am. J. Obstet. Gynecol. 148:274, 1984.

Perkins RP: Perinatal observations in a high-risk population managed without intrapartum fetal pH studies. Am. J. Obstet. Gynecol. 149:327, 1984.

Suidan JS, Young BK: Outcome of fetuses with lactic acidemia. Am. J. Obstet. Gynecol. 150:33, 1984.

Clark SL, Paul RH: Intrapartum fetal surveillance: The role of fetal scalp blood sampling. Am. J. Obstet. Gynecol. 153:717, 1985.

Breech Delivery

Collea JV, Chein C, Quilligan EJ: The randomized management of term frank breech presentation: A study of 208 cases. Am. J. Obstet. Gynecol. 137:235, 1980.

Schutterman IB, Grimes DA: Comparative safety of the low transverse versus the low vertical uterine incision for cesarean delivery of breech infants. Obstet. Gynecol. 61:593, 1983.

Tatum RK, Orr JW, Soong S, et al: Vaginal breech delivery of selected infants weighing more than 2000 grams: A retrospective analysis of seven years' experience. Am. J. Obstet. Gynecol. 152:145, 1985.

Rosen M, Debanne S, Thompson K, et al: Long-term neurological morbidity in breech and vertex births. Am. J. Obstet. Gynecol. 151:718, 1985.

Management of the breech presentation. ACOG Tech. Bull. 95, August, 1986.

Myers SA, Gleicher N: Breech delivery: Why the dilemma? Am. J. Obstet. Gynecol. 155:6, 1986.

Flanagan TA, Mulchahey KM, Korenbrot CC, et al: Management of term breech presentation. Am. J. Obstet. Gynecol. 156:1492, 1987.

Midforceps Delivery or Vacuum Extraction

Healy DL, Quinn MA, Pepperell RJ: Rotational delivery of the fetus: Kielland's forceps and two other methods compared. Br. J. Obstet. Gynaecol. 89:501, 1982.

Richardson DA, Evans MI, Cibils LA: Midforceps delivery: A critical review. Am. J. Obstet. Gynecol. 145:621, 1983.

Dierker LJ, Rosen MG, Thompson K, et al: The midforceps: Maternal and neonatal outcomes. Am. J. Obstet. Gynecol. 152:176, 1985.

Dell DL, Sightler SE, Plauche WC: Soft cup vacuum extraction: A comparison of outlet delivery. Obstet. Gynecol. 66:624, 1985.

Berkus MD, Ramamurthy RS, O'Connor PS, et al: Cohort study of silastic obstetric vacuum cup deliveries: II. Unsucccessful vacuum extraction. Obstet. Gynecol. 68:662, 1986.

Boyd ME, Usher RH, McLean FH, et al: Failed forceps. Obstet. Gynecol. 68:779, 1986.

Broekhuizen FF, Washington JM, Johnson F, et al: Vacuum extraction versus forceps delivery: Indications and complications, 1979 to 1984. Obstet. Gynecol. 69:338, 1987.

Prolapse of the Umbilical Cord

Brandeberry KR, Kistner RW: Prolapse of the umbilical cord: An analysis of 116 cases at the Cincinnati General Hospital. Am. J. Obstet. Gynecol. 61:356, 1951.

Clark DO, Copeland W, Ullery JC: Prolapse of the umbilical cord - A study of 117 cases. Am. J. Obstet. Gynecol. 101:84, 1968.

Lange LR, Manning FA, Morrison I, et al: Cord prolapse: Is antenatal diagnosis possible? Am. J. Obstet. Gynecol. 151:1083, 1985.

Emergency Cesarean Section

Gleicher N: Cesarean section rates in the United States. The short-term failure of the National Consensus Development Conference in 1980. J. Am. Med. Assoc. 252:3273, 1984.

De Regt RH, Minkoff HL, Feldman J, et al: Relation of private or clinic care to the cesarean birth rate. N. Engl. J. Med. 315:619, 1986.

Notzon FC, Placek PJ, Taffel SM: Comparisons of national cesarean-section rates. N. Engl. J. Med. 316:386, 1987.

Spellacy WN, Peterson PQ, Winnegar A, et al: Neonatal seizures after cesarean delivery: Higher risk with labor. Am. J. Obstet. Gynecol. 157:377, 1987.

Lyon JB, Richardson AC: Careful surgical technique can reduce infectious morbidity after cesarean section. Am. J. Obstet. Gynecol. 157:557, 1987.

Shoulder Dystocia

Benedetti TJ, Gabbe SG: Shoulder dystocia: A complication of fetal macrosomia and prolonged second stage of labor with midpelvic delivery. Obstet. Gynecol. 52:526, 1978.

Modanlou HD, Komatsu G, Dorchester W, et al: Large-for-gestational-age neonates: Anthropometric reasons for shoulder dystocia. Obstet. Gynecol. 60:417, 1982.

Acker DB, Sachs BP, Friedman EA: Risk factors for shoulder dystocia. Obstet. Gynecol. 66:762, 1985.

Acker DB, Sachs BP, Friedman EA: Risk factors for shoulder dystocia in the average-weight infant. Obstet. Gynecol. 67:614, 1986.

Gross SJ, Shime J, Farine D: Shoulder dystocia: Predictors and outcome. Am. J. Obstet. Gynecol. 156:334, 1987.

Gross TL, Sokol RJ, Williams T, et al: Shoulder dystocia: A fetal-physician risk. Am. J. Obstet. Gynecol. 156:1408, 1987.

Preparation for the Compromised Infant

Paneth N, Stark RI: Cerebral palsy and mental retardation in relation to indicators of perinatal asphyxia: An epidemiologic overview. Am. J. Obstet. Gynecol. 147:960, 1983.

Rayburn WF, Donn SM, Kolin MG, et al: Obstetric care and intraventricular hemorrhage in the low birth weight infant. Obstet. Gynecol. 61:408, 1983.

Tejani N, Rebold B, Tuck S, et al: Obstetric factors in the causation of early periventricular-intraventricular hemorrhage. Obstet. Gynecol. 64:510, 1984.

Nelson KB, Ellenberg JH: Obstetric complications as risk factors for cerebral palsy or seizure disorders. J. Am. Med. Asso. 251:1843, 1984.

Levine MG, Holroyde J, Woods JR, et al: Birth trauma: Incidence and predisposing factors. Obstet. Gynecol. 63:792, 1984.

Keegan KA, Waffarn F, Quilligan EJ: Obstetric characteristics and fetal heart rate patterns of infants who convulse during the newborn period. Am. J. Obstet. Gynecol. 153:732, 1985.

Low JA, Galbraith RS, Muir DW, et al: The relationship between perinatal hypoxia and newborn encephalopathy. Am. J. Obstet. Gynecol. 152:256, 1985.

Dijxhoorn MJ, Visser GHA, Fidler VJ, et al: Apgar score, meconium and acidaemia at birth in relation to neonatal neurological morbidity in term infants. Br. J. Obstet. Gynaecol. 93:217, 1986.

Shankaran S, Cepeda EE, Ilagan N, et al: Antenatal phenobarbital for the prevention of neonatal intracerebral hemorrhage. Am. J. Obstet. Gynecol. 154:53, 1986.

Nelson KB, Ellenberg JH: Antecedents of cerebral palsy. Multivariate analysis of risk. N. Engl. J. Med. 315:81, 1986.

Morales WJ, Koerten J: Prevention of intraventricular hemorrhage in very low birth weight infants by maternally administered phenobarbital. Obstet. Gynecol. 68:295, 1986.

Paul RH, Yonekura L, Cantrell CJ, et al: Fetal injury prior to labor: Does it happen? Am. J. Obstet. Gynecol. 154:1187, 1986.

Hensleigh PA, Fainstat T, Spencer R: Perinatal events and cerebral palsy. Am. J. Obstet. Gynecol. 154:978, 1986.

Rosen MG, Hobel CJ: Prenatal and perinatal factors associated with brain disorders. Obstet. Gynecol. 68:416, 1986.

Patriarcco MS, Viechnicki BM, Hutchinson TA, et al: A study on intrauterine fetal resuscitation with terbutaline. Am. J. Obstet. Gynecol. 157:384, 1987.

Chapter 10

Postpartum Care

Postpartum Hemorrhage

The most commonly accepted definition of postpartum hemorrhage is a blood loss in excess of 500 ml in the immediate postpartum period. However, when blood loss has been measured carefully, the following findings have been observed consistently: 1) the average blood loss with vaginal delivery is approximately 600 ml, 2) only about 5% of women hemorrhage more than 1,000 ml, and 3) the estimated blood loss is often approximately half of the carefully measured blood loss. An awareness of risk factors enumerated in Table 10.1 should allow anticipation of most cases of postpartum hemorrhage.

All hospitalized patients should have their blood type and screen performed before delivery. Early and aggressive management prevents hemorrhage from becoming life-threatening and decreases the likelihood of complications from anemia. The early establishment of personal contact with blood bank personnel is encouraged.

Table 10.1
Conditions Predisposing to Postpartum Hemorrhage

Multiparity of more than five babies	Prolonged labor
Previous postpartum hemorrhage or manual removal of the placenta	Precipitous labor
	Difficult forceps delivery
Abruptio placentae	Version and extraction
Placenta previa	Chorioamnionitis
Excessive inhalational anesthesia	Breech extraction
Multiple pregnancy	Cesarean section
Polyhydramnios	Excesive or prolonged
Prolonged retention of a dead fetus	oxytocin administration

Prophylaxis

1. A hematocrit should be determined during labor, and blood should be sent for type and screening.
2. When hemorrhage is anticipated, 2 units of blood should be cross-matched and available. A red top tube of blood should be tested for a prolonged clotting time (beyond 5 min) for possible transfusion.
3. Fibrinogen levels should be determined in cases of a large placental abruption, retained dead fetus, severe preeclampsia, or eclampsia.
4. Unless rapid delivery is imperative, the fetus and placenta should be delivered slowly to allow the uterus to contract sufficiently.
5. In cases where uterine atony is anticipated, intravenous oxytocin (10-40 units/liter IVF) added after delivery is continued for at least 1 hr postpartum.
6. Careful postpartum observation is necessary, and the uterine fundus should be massaged frequently for at least 1 hr postpartum.

Supportive Measures

1. In the presence of excessive bleeding, manual removal of the placenta should be carried out promptly. Voluntary pushing by the mother to expel the placenta out may be helpful. Another physician should assist, while blood is set up for possible transfusion.
2. Careful inspection of the genital tract is necessary with adequate lighting. An assistant is an invaluable asset.
3. General anesthesia should be discontinued, and oxygen should be given by face mask.
4. Until blood is available, plasma expanders such as Lactated Ringer's or normal saline are used. A minimum of 1 liter of packed red blood cells or whole blood should be transfused.
5. If the blood pressure is falling, the foot of the table should be elevated.
6. Uterine atony is the most common reason for persistent postpartum bleeding. Uterine massage and compression of the aorta are recommended. Other causes of hemorrhage to be considered are listed in Table 10.2.
7. Transfusion with platelets, cryoprecipitate, or fresh frozen plasma is rarely necessary. Coagulation studies (PTT, PT, platelet count) should be performed beforehand. If hypofibrinogenemia is present, fibrinogen in cryoprecipitate (usually 10-20 packs) or fresh frozen plasma (usually 4 units) should be administered intravenously. If severe thrombocytopenia ($20,000/mm^2$ or less) exists, 6-10 packs of platelets should be infused to raise the platelet count by $15-60,000/mm^2$.
8. An ultrasound examination of the uterine cavity to look for retained placental fragments may be useful during immediate or delayed postpartum hemorrhage.

Table 10.2
Causes of Postpartum Hemorrhage

Uterine atony
Retained placental fragment
Cervical or vaginal tear
Paravaginal, vulvar, or broad ligament hematoma
Intraperitoneal bleeding from a ruptured uterus
Afibrinogenemia, hypofibrinogenemia, thrombocytopenia, or
 inadequate platelet aggregation
Septic shock
Uterine inversion

Blood Component Replacement

Packed Red Blood Cells

Red blood cells provide a source of oxygen-carrying erythrocytes and mass for volume replacement. All units of blood are routinely screened for hepatitis B antigen and HIV antibody. Side effects and hazards (immunization, febrile reaction, iron overload, allergic reaction, hemolysis) of PRBC transfusion are similar but less severe than from whole blood, since plasma, metabolites, and antibodies are removed. The typical red blood cell unit contains 200 ml of erythrocytes (hematocrit 70-80%), which should raise the recipient's hematocrit by 3%. When combined with isotonic saline, the transfusion of a unit should not exceed 4 hours. Infrequent side effects or hazards include hypokalemia with massive transfusion and microaggregates of fibrin, platelets, and white blood cells that would not be retained in the ordinary blood filter.

Platelets

Platelet concentrates, derived from donor blood, are used in patients with thrombocytopenia unless rapid platelet destruction is evident. Immunization to red blood cell antigens is possible because of the presence of a small number of red blood cells in the platelet packs. Therefore, prevention of $Rh_o(D)$ sensitization may require Rh immune globulin when an Rh negative woman is transfused by an Rh positive donor.

One unit of platelets usually increases the platelet count by $5,000-10,000/mm^2$. The usual dose of a 10-unit pack is given when bleeding symptoms are evident or a platelet count is below $20,000/mm^2$. Repeat transfusion may be required because the half-life of platelets is only 3-4 days.

Fresh Frozen Plasma

Fresh frozen plasma is separated from a donor's blood within 6 hours after collection. It is an excellent source of the clotting factors V, VII, IX, and fibrinogen. The typical unit contains 225-275 ml of anticoagulated plasma with 200 units of factor VIII, 200 units of factor IX, and 400 mg of fibrinogen. As with cryoprecipitate, donor compatibility is unimportant, but antibodies within the plasma can react to the recipient cells.

Cryoprecipitate
Cryoprecipitate, a source of the coagulation factors VIII, XIII, and fibrinogen, is used for hemophilia A, hypofibrinogenemia, and von Willebrand's disease. As with other plasma products, viral hepatitis may be transmitted and febrile allergic reactions may occur. The amount of these factors required for adequate coagulation is not easily predictable and varies with the clinical situation. Like fresh frozen plasma, cryoprecipitate is usually transported from a community facility, then thawed and kept at room temperature for up to 6 hrs before use.

Treatment of Uterine Atony

Along with vigorous uterine massage and aortic compression, the following measures may be taken to control excess bleeding from presumed uterine atony.

Ergonovine	Ergonovine maleate (Methergine) 0.2 mg is given intravenously or intramuscularly (unless hypertension is already present).
Oxytocin	20-40 units of oxytocin in a liter of intravenous fluids at a speed sufficient to keep the uterus contracted.
Uterine exploration	Blood clots and placental fragments are removed.
Lacerations	The cervix, vagina, and vulva are examined and repaired with proper lighting and exposure by an assistant.
Uterine compression	One hand is placed in the vagina against the lower anterior wall of the uterus. The uterus is sharply anteflexed. Massaging pressure is exerted against the anteflexed aspect of the uterus by the other hand on the abdomen. A catheter in the bladder is helpful.
Prostaglandins	The vaginal insertion of a prostaglandin E_2 suppository (20 mg) with a vaginal pack or the intramuscular or myometrial injection of prostaglandin F_{2alpha} (1 ml) in the buttock may be useful if treatment using oxytocin or ergonovine is unsuccessful. Additional doses may be necessary.

Uterine packing or warm saline lavage	Most authorities condemn its use, since these procedures are not physiologic. One or two 5- or 10-yard rolls of gauze are packed tightly first into one corner of the uterus and then the other.
Intrauterine curetting	Unless placental fragments are palpable, curetting using a "banjo" currette is not usually beneficial.
Ligation of uterine arteries	The abdomen is opened, the uterus is elevated by the surgeon's hand, and the area of the uterine vessels in the lower broad ligament is exposed. Using a large needle and no. 1 chromic catgut or vicryl suture, a stitch is placed through a substantial part of the lower segment of the myometrium, 2-3 cm medial to the vessels. The vessels are ligated but not divided. Subsequent menstruation and pregnancy are usually unaffected.
Ligation of hypogastric arteries	The common iliac artery and its bifurcation into the external and internal iliac (hypogastric) arteries are palpated and visualized through the posterior peritoneum. The ureter crosses anterior to the bifurcation of the common iliac artery, and it must be identified to prevent potential damage. The posterior peritoneum is tented and incised in a longitudinal direction at the level of the origin of the internal iliac artery, lateral to the ureter and medial to the internal iliac artery. Two no. 2-0 silk sutures are placed around the internal iliac artery 1 cm apart and then tied on each side.
Angiographic embolization	A competent angiographer may be able to selectively embolize the uterine or hypogastric arteries with Gelfoam fragments. Subsequent menstruation, fertility, and pregnancy are usually unaffected.
Hysterectomy	If the above measures are ineffective, a hysterectomy should be performed. Deaths following and during hysterectomy usually result from delaying the operation until the patient is nearly moribund.

Postpartum Infection

Postpartum infectious morbidity is considered to be present when a parturient experiences a fever of ≥38 C (100.4 F) on two occasions or more during the first 10 postpartum days, exclusive of the first 24 hrs. The incidence of febrile morbidity varies widely, ranging from approximately 1% for nonindigent women delivering vaginally to as high as 87% for indigent women delivering by cesarean section. Factors definitely identified as increasing the risk of infection include emergency cesarean section, labor, ruptured membranes for 6 hrs or more, and low socioeconomic status. Other factors such as anemia, general anesthesia, poor nutrition, obesity, and multiple vaginal exams may influence the risk of infection, but the correlation is less firmly established. All other factors being equal, the use of internal fetal monitoring does not appear to influence the risk of uterine infection.

The differential for postpartum infection should include the seven W's: womb, wound, wind (atelectasis, pneumonia), water (urinary tract), wonder drug (drug allergy), walk (thrombophlebitis), and woman's breasts (bacterial and noninfectious mastitis). Most febrile morbidity results from an infection of the genital tract which is usually polymicrobial and frequently involves anaerobic organisms (Bacteroides fragilis, Peptostreptococcus). It is difficult to assess the role of transcervical cultures, because the normal resident flora of the genital tract makes interpretation of culture results difficult. The use of a double or triple-lumen lavage catheter may avoid vaginal/cervical contamination when collecting uterine specimens.

Wound and urinary tract infections are also relatively common. During evaluation of the febrile parturient, a diligent effort should be made to determine the site of infection and eliminate the less common causes of infection. Antibiotic regimens recommended to eradicate causative organisms in certain postpartum infections are shown in Table 10.3. Cure rates of endomyometritis using these regimens are expected to be 70-95%. Sequestered infections (abscess, hematoma, septic pelvic thrombophlebitis) or resistant organisms (Klebsiella, Enterococcus, nosocomial Staphyllococcus aureus) may not respond well to these regimens.

Contraceptive Counseling

Contraceptive counseling during the postpartum period is essential to educate the new mother about forms of contraception and when she may safely become sexually active. The proper contraceptive choice requires a knowledge of the patient's motivation and a knowledge of the effectiveness, safety, and convenience of the various contraceptives. Oral contraception is the most effective nonpermanent form of birth control; however, if oral contraceptives are used improperly, barrier techniques may instead provide better protection.

Table 10.3
Antibiotic Therapy for Certain Postpartum Infections

Infection/ Common Isolates	Antibiotic Regimen	Alternate Regimen
Bacteriuria Escherichia coli	Ampicillin 500 mg po qid, 7-10 days	Based on bacterial susceptibility testing
Streptococcus fecalis (enterococcus)	Ampicillin 500 mg po qid, 7-10 days	Based on bacterial susceptibility testing
Proteus mirabilis	Ampicillin 500 mg po qid, 7-10 days	Cephalexin 0.5- 1.0 gm po q 6 hr
Klebsiella spp.	Ampicillin 500 mg po qid, 7-10 days or cephalexin 0.5 gm po q 6 hr, 7-10 days	Tetracycline 500 mg po q 6 hr
Endomyometritis and postpartum sepsis Group A or B beta-hemolytic streptococcus	Penicillin G 1×10^6 units IV q 4-6 hr until afebrile for 3 days, then oral penicillin to complete 10-day course	Cefazolin 50 mg/kg/ day q 6 hr
Escherichia coli	Gentamicin 5 mg/kg/ day IV q 8 hr or ampicillin 150-200 mg/kg/day q 4 hr	Cefazolin 50 mg/kg/ day IV q 6 hr
Bacteroides fragilis	Clindamycin 20-25 mg/kg/day IV q 6 hr po or IV q 6 hr or cefoxitin 2 gm IV q 8 hr	Chloramphenicol 50-75 mg/kg/day
Undetermined	Cefoxitin 2 gm IV q 8 hr or Clindamycin 600 mg IV q 6 hr and gentamicin 1 mg/kg IV q 8 hr	Piperacillin, ticarcillin, metronidazole

Table 10.3 (Continued)

Infection/ Common Isolates	Antibiotic Regimen	Alternate Regimen
Postinstrumentation Mixed flora	Ampicillin 150-200 mg/kg/day IV q 4 hr and gentamicin 5 mg/kg/ day IV q 8 hr	Based on bacterial susceptibility testing
Pelvic abscess Mixed aerobic and anaerobic flora	Ampicillin 150-200 mg/kg/day IV q 4 hr, gentamicin 5 mg/kg/day IV q 8 hr, and clindamycin 20-25 mg/kg/day IV q 6 hr	Based on bacterial susceptibility testing
Pelvic thrombophlebitis Bacteroides spp.	Ampicillin, gentamicin, and clindamycin (along with heparin)	Cefoxitin, piperacillin, metronidazole, or ticarcillin
Pneumonia Streptococcus pneumoniae	Benzyl penicillin 1 x 10^6 units IV q 6 hr or procaine penicillin 600,000 units IM q 12 hr	Erythromycin 0.5 gm po q 6 hr
Mycoplasma pneumoniae	Erythromycin 0.5 gm po q 6 hr	Tetracycline 500 mg po or IV
Hemophilus influenza	Ampicillin 150-200 mg/kg/day IV q 6 hr	Cefamandole 500 mg po or IV
Staph. aureus	Nafcillin 150-200 mg/kg/day IV q 4 hr	Cefazolin 1 gm IV q 6 hr or clindamycin po or IV 300 mg q 6 hr
Gram-negative enteric bacilli	Gentamicin or tobramycin 5 mg/kg/day IV q 8 hr	Based on bacterial susceptibility testing
Pseudomonas aeruginosa	Ticarcillin 200-300 mg/kg/day IV q 4 hr and tobramycin 5 mg/kg/day IV q 8 hr	Based on bacterial susceptibility testing

Table 10.3 (Continued)

Infection Common Isolates	Antibiotic Regimen	Alternate Regimen
Cellulitis Staph. aureus	Nafcillin 150-200 mg/kg/day IV q 4 hr	Based on bacterial susceptibility testing
Beta-hemolytic streptococcus	Aqueous penicillin G 1×10^6 units IV q 4 hr	Cefazolin 50 mg/ kg/day IV q 6 hr

Pregnancy itself is a greater health risk than any available form of birth control. A patient who is 30 years or older has an additional mortality risk associated with oral contraceptive use and smoking. Although unacceptable to many, a barrier method of contraception backed up by abortion is perhaps the safest method of contraception at any age and has a 100% effectiveness. First year contraceptive failure rates for reproductive age women are listed in Table 10.4.

Oral Contraceptives

Before beginning a patient on oral contraceptives, the physician should be aware of absolute and relative contraindications as listed in Table 10.5. Certain drugs interact with oral contraceptives by either reducing the contraceptive efficacy or by modifying the activities of the drug. Management changes to reduce drug interactions are proposed in Table 10.6.

When to Start the Pill after Delivery

Initiation of oral contraceptive therapy depends on the time of delivery. A patient may be started on an oral contraceptive immediately after pregnancy termination at 12 weeks or less. Because of the added risk of thrombus formation in the postpartum period, a

Table 10.4
First Year Contraceptive Failure Rates

Form of Contraception	Pregnancies/Year/100 Users
Sterilization	0.1-0.4
Oral contraceptives	2
Condoms	10
Diaphragm	13
Foam, cream, jelly	15
Rhythm	19
All others	11

Table 10.5
Absolute (A) and Relative (R) Contraindications to Oral
Contraceptive Use

_____

Vascular
   A   Phlebitis
   A   Pulmonary embolus
   A   Cerebral vascular acccident
   A   Coronary occlusion
   A   Blood dyscrasias - leukemia, sickle cell anemia, and poly-
       cythemia are associated with intravascular blood clotting

Liver
   A   Jaundice - chronic or recurrent
   A   Hepatitis - active or chronic with decreased liver function
   R   Recurrent pruritis of pregnancy
   A   Cirrhosis with decreased liver function
   A   Hepatic prophyria
   A   Hepatic tumor

Metabolic
   R   Predisposition to diabetes mellitus (direct family history,
       family history and obesity, history of macrosomic infant(s)
       or gestational diabetes)
   A   Hypertension (documented blood pressure 140/90 or higher or
       separate occasions)
   R   Previous history of high blood pressure
   R   Black, with family history of high blood pressure
   A   Lipids (increased triglycerides, age 38 and over)

Reproduction
   A   Pregnanccy
   R   Breast feeding
   A 1^0 amenorrhea
   A 2^0 amenorrhea - history of repeated cessation of menstrual
       periods for 3 or more months or chronic infrequent periods
   R 2^0 amenorrhea or lactation while on OCs - cessation of
       menstrual periods and/or breast discharge
   R   Chronic breakthrough bleeding on OCs - unpredictable
       bleeding while on OCs
   A   Chronic cystic mastitis in smoker

Miscellaneous Concurrent Diseases
   R   Epilepsy
   A   Migraine headaches
   A   Prophyria
   R   Fibroid tumors of uterus
   R   Benign breast tumors
   A   Varicose veins - severe
   R   Gallstones or chronic biliary symptoms
   A   Hyperthyroidism
   R   Diabetes mellitus
   A   Malignant neoplastic disease

Table 10.6
Drugs That Interact with Oral Contraceptives

Drug	Presumed Mechanism of Action	Suggested Management
Drugs That May Reduce the Efficacy of Oral Contraceptives		
Anticonvulsants		
Barbiturates Phenobarbital Primidone Phenytoin	Fluid retention caused by OCs may precipitate seizures; induction of microsomal liver enzymes	20-35 mcg combination OCs or progestin only pills or another method
Phenylbutazone and allied drugs		
Phenylbutazone Indomethacin Ibuprofen	Hepatic microsomal enzyme induction	Use alternate method
Antibiotics		
Rifampicin Penicillin	Enzyme induction; rapid breakdown of estrogen in liver; intestinal motility increased with penicillins	Higher-dose OCs during short course of antibiotics or additional contraceptives; for long course, use another method
Sedatives and hypnotics		
Benzodiazepines Barbiturates	Enzyme induction; increased estrogen metabolism	Alternative method
Modification of Other Drug Activity by Oral Contraceptives		
Anticoagulants	Efficacy impaired, as OCs increase clotting factors	Do no use OCs with anticoagulant therapy
Antidiabetic agents		
Insulin and oral hypoglycemic agents	High-dose estrogen pills cause impaired glucose tolerance	Use 20-35 mcg OCs or progestin only; consider other methods
Antihypertensives		
Guanethidine and occasionally methyldopa	Estrogen component involved with sodium retention and increased angiotensinogen	Use progestin-only pill or another method
Phenothiazines		
All phenothiazines Reserpine, tricyclic	Serum prolactin altered, while combination OCs are associated with increased serum prolactin levels to TRH	Use alternative method

patient who delivers after 12 weeks should usually wait at least three weeks before beginning oral contraceptives.

If she wishes to nurse while taking oral contraceptives, the pills should be started several days after delivery, and a low-dose estrogen pill should be prescribed so as not to interfere with milk production or quality.

Selection of the Proper Pill

The estrogen and progestin components should be considered when selecting the proper pill. Listed in Table 10.7 are a few of the more than 30 oral contraceptive brands. The first choice of oral contraception should contain a low-dose estrogen component to minimize risks. The preparation may be changed to a more intermediate dose if menstrual problems (spotting, etc.) are not resolved after a usual three month trial. A combination pill with a mildly androgenic progestin component is also desirable. High dose combination pills are rarely if ever indicated.

Patient Concerns

Once the pill is begun, the patient should use a second contraceptive method such as foam and condoms for the first menstrual cycle, even though the birth control pill should be nearly 100% effective within a few days after starting. An adequate trial of the preparation should last 3 months before changing to a different preparation or discontinuing the pill. Many minor side effects can be ameliorated by switching formulations within the same estrogen range.

There is no apparent need to discontinue the oral contraceptive for a "rest period," since a high incidence of unwanted pregnancies is associated with this practice. The decision to discontinue the birth control pill for a planned pregnancy should include a minimum of one menstrual cycle before conception after discontinuing the pills. This will permit a more accurate determination of the estimated date of confinement.

Certain side effects may arise from the use of oral contraceptives. These include menstrual abnormalities, gastrointestinal disturbances, central nervous system symptoms, and endocrine organ problems. Listed in Table 10.8 are frequent patient concerns and recommended therapy.

Some of the most important research in recent years has established health benefits from oral contraceptive exposure. There is thought to be a decreased risk of the following: benign breast lesions (fibroadenomas and fibrocystic disease), ovarian tumors (benign and malignant), endometrial carcinoma, endometriosis, pelvic inflammatory disease, dysmenorrhea and premenstrual symptoms. Menstrual cycles would also be better regulated with less menorrhagia.

Table 10.7
Common Oral Contraceptive Brands

More Estrogenic	Intermediate	More Androgenic
Low Dose Demulen 1/35	Brevicon, Modicon, Nordette Loestrin 1/20, Zorane 1/20 OrthoNovum 1/35 Ovcon 35, Triphasil Ortho- Novum 7, 7, 7	Lo/Ovral
Intermediate Dose Demulen	OrthoNovum 1/50, Norinyl 1/50, Ovcon 50	Ovral
High Dose Ovulen	OrthoNovum 2 mg Norlestrin 2.5 mg	Ovral 1/80

Diaphragm

A diaphragm should not usually be fitted until at least 1 month after delivery. At that time the patient should be instructed on its proper fit such that the lower edge is around the cervix, and the upper edge is posterior to the pubic arc. The patient's ability to properly insert and remove the diaphragm should be checked before she leaves the clinic. Once the patient has been able to comfortably insert and remove the diaphragm, she should be instructed on using an additional form of contraception (foam, condoms) during the initial month as she becomes better acccustomed to the use of a diaphragm with spermicidal jelly.

The diaphragm should be inserted no more than 6 hrs before coitus and left in place for at least 8 hrs after coitus. Additional spermicide is necessary for each coitus before the diaphragm is removed. Refitting of the diaphragm is necessary if there is a weight change in excess of 10 pounds, pelvic discomfort, difficulty in micturition, or delivery after a recent pregnancy. The diaphragm should be inspected periodically for any perforations.

Condoms

When used properly and with an awareness of the woman's menstrual cycle, the condom method of birth control is theoretically quite effective. However, improper use is associated with a failure rate of approximately 10-15%, and a spermicidal gel or foam is often recommended in addition to the condom to improve its effectiveness.

Spermicidal Agents

The spermicidal agent in all vaginal foams, suppositories, and creams is nonoxynol-9 in sufficient concentration to effectively kill sperm and to act as a barrier between the sperm and cervical canal.

Table 10.8
Undesired Effects from Oral Contraceptives

Problem	Recommendations
Hyperandrogenism (acne, hirsutism, weight gain)	Change to less androgenic progestin compound
Breast (mastodynia, enlargement)	Use lower dose estrogen/progestin (progestin should be more androgenic) i.e., Lo Ovral or Ovral
Amenorrhea	Rule out pregnancy Discontinue pills for 3 months if worrisome to patient Recycle with higher-dose estrogen component
Postpill amenorrhea	Hormone profile (FSH, LH, Prl) Cycle with an estrogen (Premarin 1.25 mcg) for days 1-25 and a progestin (Provera 10 mg) for days 15-25. Ovulation stimulation (Clomid) after hormone profile if pregnancy desired
Amenorrhea-galactorrhea	Serum prolactin Rule out pituitary tumor Pap smear of any unilateral breast discharge Discontinue pills
Premenstrual tension (fluid retention, nervous, irritable, headache)	Use lower dose estrogen/progestin preparation Sodium restricted diet Minimize use of diuretics Pyridoxine 30 mg QID
Breakthrough bleeding (BTB) beyond 3rd cycle	Use higher dose estrogen/progestin preparation If BTB continues, discontinue pills Consider dilation and curettage if persists.
Chloasma	Use minimal dose estrogen/progestin preparation Avoid exposure to sunlight
CNS symptoms (fatigue, lassitude, decreased libido, mild depression, headaches)	Use low-dose estrogen/progestin Multiple vitamin replacement Pyridoxine 30 mg QID (?) Take pill at night or discontinue if persists

Table 10.8 (Continued)

Problem	Recommendations
GI disturbances (nausea, vomiting, epigastric distress, bloating, pruritis)	Use low-dose estrogen/progestin preparation Pruritis associated with BSP retention and occcasional peripheral bile salts; therapy with oral cholestyramine and discontinue OCs Take pill at night or discontinue if persists
Monilial vaginitis	Monilial treatment, consider more estrogenic preparation Discontinue pill if persists Screen for glucose intolerance

Vaginal spermicides should not be used as the sole contraceptive technique. They may be useful in particular with an unplanned coitus, immediately postpartum, or in women over 40 years of age.

The agent should be placed as close to the vaginal apex and cervix as possible within 1 hr before coitus. Douching is contraindicated for at least 8 hrs after intercourse. Additional spermicide should be reapplied before each coitus. If a suppository is used, a delay of 10 min from suppository insertion to coitus is recommended. If foam is used, the container should be shaken well, and a second container should be available.

The vaginal contraceptive sponge has been marketed since 1983 and is a relatively expensive method of birth control. Clinical trials with vaginal sponges containing a spermicidal agent suggest a contraceptive effectiveness comparable to the diaphragm as both mechanical and clinical sperm barriers are employed.

Rhythm Method

The rhythm method alone is often inadequate for contraception. However, it may be a useful technique in select patients with regular menstrual cycles who are between planned pregnancies or in women who do not wish to use another form of contraception. The ovum is capable of being fertilized within 48 hrs after ovulation, and the sperm are capable of fertilizing the ovum for 24 hrs after ejaculation. Therefore, the fertile period during each cycle is extended 3 days in which the ovum is capable of being fertilized.

A thorough knowledge of her menstrual cycle pattern is imperative if a woman is to be able to predict the time of ovulation with reasonable certainty. Some women are aware of an increase in vaginal discharge or change in cervical mucous texture near mid-cycle which can be helpful indicators of ovulation. A basal body temperature graph is useful in determining a 0.5-1° F temperature elevation following ovulation because of the thermogenic properties of progesterone. Abstinence from coital activity for at least 3 days after the sustained elevation in temperature is necessary to increase the effectiveness of the rhythm method.

Counseling the Teenager

An unwanted teenage pregnancy is associated with multiple psychologic and medical sequelae which include an increased rate of therapeutic abortion, medical complications of pregnancy, enrollment in the welfare system, failure to complete high school, divorce, child abuse or neglect, and suicide. The oral contraceptive is often preferred, since barrier techniques require patient motivation and education. A low-dose oral contraceptive is recommended with the progestin component being other than norgestrel (too androgenic). Most side effects from oral contraceptive use relate directly to the estrogen dosage, so the lower dose preparations are less likely to cause breast discomfort, breakthrough bleeding, nausea, or fluid retention. The 28-pill packet may be preferred to improve patient compliance.

Ideally, the teenager should not begin oral contraceptives until well after her delivery and only after spontaneous menstrual cycles with predicted intervals have been reestablished. However, it must be remembered that ovulation may occur as soon as 2 weeks after abortion and 4 weeks after a term delivery.

Future Contraceptive Alternatives

A nonpermanent form of birth control should be effective, safe, and reversible. Contraceptives that may become commercially available in the next few years include the cervical cap (a rubber cap that fits around the cervix and is left in place several days) and subdermal hormone rods or capsules which inhibit ovulation for up to 7 yrs. Long-range birth control possibilities which require further research and clinical refinement include hormone-releasing vaginal rings (work like oral contraceptives and remain in place for 3-4 wks), disposable diaphragms (contain a spermicide that is effective for 24 hrs), long-acting norethindrone enanthate injections (inhibit ovulation for 60-90 days), longer acting vaginal suppositories (12-16 hrs compared with 2 hrs), LHRH analogs (when injected or implanted may inhibit sperm production), and immunizations against sperm antibodies or hCG.

Postpartum Hypertension

Elevations in blood pressures among patients with pregnancy-induced hypertension will usually return to a normotensive range within a few days after delivery. The likelihood for developing essential hypertension later in adulthood is highly variable (2-60%), but probably is not increased unless there is residual hypertension, renal impairment, or preexisting hypertension.

Any patient whose blood pressure remains elevated during the first three postpartum days should be managed expectantly with intermittent, parenteral hydralazine (5-15 mg) given if the diastolic is 105 mm Hg or higher. If tachycardia is present, clonidine (Catapres) may be used instead. A search for signs of central nervous system irritability is also important since eclampsia can occur as long as one week postpartum.

If blood presure values remain elevated after the third postpartum day, the following measures should be undertaken: a) consider the family dynamics, especially the patient's reaction to her newborn infant, b) begin to evaluate renal function (creatinine clearance, urine protein), c) instruct the patient on self blood pressure monitoring, and d) if blood pressures are borderline (140-150/90-100), sedate with phenobarbital 30 mg BID-QID. If diastolic values are more than 100, begin diuretic therapy (ex. hydrochlorothiazide 50 mg daily or bid). Although less commonly used, methyldopa or a beta-blocker such as atenolol or labetalol have also been used successfully.

Unless normotensive within a few days after delivery, the patient should be reexamined in the clinic in 1 week. If the blood pressure remains elevated, an appointment should be made with an internist for diagnostic evaluation and possible antihypertensive therapy.

A low-dose oral contraceptive may be prescribed at the 6-week postpartum visit if the patient is normotensive and temporary contraceptive methods do not fit the patient's needs. Blood pressure should continue to be monitored on a regular basis.

Drugs in Breast Milk

The prevalence of breast feeding has increased dramatically during the past decade coinciding with an avoidance of artificial products and processes. The importance of maternal-infant bonding during the early newborn period is often emphasized by health care professionals, and many women try to breast feed at least during the initial postpartum period. It is important to be aware that breast milk can be a significant source of infant drug exposure, and weaning as a precaution requires accurate information about the drug level in breast milk and its effect on the infant.

Under most circumstances, the quantity of a drug or chemical excreted in the milk is quite low, with milk levels being less than maternal serum levels. Any effect on the infant is usually not significant unless maternal therapy is prolonged or in higher than therapeutic doses or if the infant is premature. Unacceptably high drug concentrations may be found in milk when isoniazid, metronidazole, nitrofurantoin, and sulfa preparations are prescribed. Neonatal effects at therapeutic doses in the mother are shown in Appendix A.2.

Suggested Readings

Postpartum Hemorrhage

Watson P, Besch N, Bowes WA: Management of acute and subacute puerperal inversion of the uterus. Obstet. Gynecol. 55:12, 1980.

Clark SL, Yeh SY, Phelan JP, et al: Emergency hysterectomy for obstetric hemorrhage. Obstet. Gynecol. 64:376, 1984.

Hemorrhagic shock. ACOG Tech. Bull. 82, December, 1984.

Blood component therapy. ACOG Tech. Bull. 78, July, 1984.

Hayashi RH, Castillo MS, Noah ML: Management of severe postpartum hemorrhage with a prostaglandin F_2 alpha-analogue. Obstet. Gynecol. 63:806, 1984.

Evans S, McShane P: The efficacy of internal iliac artery ligation in obstetric hemorrhage. Surg. Gynecol. Obstet. 160:250, 1985.

Postpartum Infection

Gibbs RS, Rodgers PJ, Castaneda YS, et al: Endometritis following vaginal delivery. Obstet. Gynecol. 56:555, 1980.

Sweet RL, Yonekura ML, Hill G, et al: Appropriate use of antibiotics in serious obstetric and gynecologic infections. Am. J. Obstet. Gynecol. 146:719, 1983.

Nielsen TF, Hokegard K: Postoperative cesarean section morbidity: A prospective study. Am. J. Obstet. Gynecol. 146:911, 1983.

Thomsen AC, Espersen T, Maigaard S: Course and treatment of milk stasis, noninfectious inflammation of the breast, and infectious mastitis in nursing women. Am. J. Obstet. Gynccol. 149:492, 1984.

Hurry DJ, Larsen B, Charles D: Effects of postcesarean section febrile morbidity on subsequent fertility. Obstet. Gynecol. 64:256, 1984.

Duff P: Pathophysiology and management of postcesarean endomyometritis. Obstet. Gynecol. 67:269, 1986.

Contraceptive Counseling

Hilgers TW, Abraham GE, Cavanagh D: Natural family planning I. The peak symptom and estimated time of ovulation. Am. J. Obstet. Gynecol. 52:575, 1978.

Faich G, Pearson K, Fleming D, et al: Toxic shock syndrome and the vaginal contraceptive sponge. J. Am. Med. Asso. 225:216, 1986.

Powell MG, Mears BJ, Deber RB, et al: Contraception with the cervical cap: Effectiveness, safety, continuity of use, and user satisfaction. Contraception 33:215, 1986.

McIntyre SL, Higgins JE: Parity and use-effectiveness with the contraceptive sponge. Am. J. Obstet. Gynecol. 155:796, 1986.

Oral contraception. ACOG Tech. Bull. 106, July, 1987.

International Symposium on Contraception. Am. J. Obstet. Gynecol. 157:1019-1092, 1987.

Postpartum Hypertension

Drugs for hypertension. Medical Letter 29:1, January, 1987.

Kirshon B, Lee W, Cotton D, et al: Indirect blood pressure monitoring in the postpartum patient. Obstet. Gynecol. 70:799, 1987.

Appendix 1

A.1 Drug Effects on the Human Fetus

Drug	First Trimester Effects	Second & Third Trimester Effects
Analgesics		
Acetaminophen	None known	Nephrotoxicity (?)
Narcotics	None known	Depression, withdrawal
Salicylates	None proven	Prolonged pregnancy and labor, hemorrhage, closure of ductus arteriosus (?)
Anesthetics		
General	Anomalies abortion	Depression
Local	None known	Bradycardia seizures
Anorexics		
Amphetamines	Possible cardiac defects	Irritability, poor feeding
Phenmetrazine	Skeletal anomalies (?)	None known
Meclazine	Facial cleft (?)	None known
Anti-infection Agents		
Aminoglycosides	Possible nerve and renal anomalies	Nephrotoxic, ototoxic
Ampicillin	None known	None known
Cephalosporins	None known	None known
Chloramphenicol	None known	"Gray baby" syndrome (?)
Clindamycin	None known	Unknown
Erythromycin	None known	None known
Ethambutol	None known	None known
Ethionamide	Anomalies	None known
Isoniazid	None known	None known
Metronidazole	Mutagenesis (?); no increase in anom.	None known
Nitrofurantoin	None known	Hemolytic anemia (?)
Penicillins	None known	None known
Rifampin	None known	None known
Sulfonamides	None known	Hemolytic anemia, thrombocytopenia hyperbilirubinemia
Streptomycin	Hearing deficit	Hearing deficit, VIII nerve damage

A.1 (Continued)

Drugs	First Trimester Effects	Second & Third Trimester Effects
Tetracyclines	Impaired bone growth	Stained deciduous teeth (enamel hypoplasia); impaired limb development (?)
Trimethaprim	None known (theoretic concern)	Hyperbilirubinemia
Anticoagulants		
Coumadin	Nasal hypoplasia, ophthalmic abnormalities, epiphyseal stippling	Hemorrhage, stillbirth, mental retardation, optic atrophy, microcephaly
Heparin	None known	Hemorrhage, stillbirth
Anticonvulsants		
Barbiturates	None known	Bleeding, withdrawal
Carbamazepine	Unknown	Bleeding, withdrawal
Clonazepam	None known	Withdrawal, depression
Ethosuximide	None known	None known
Phenytoin	IUGR, craniofacial abnormalities, mental retardation, hypoplasia of phalanges	Hemorrhage (depletion of vitamin K-dependent clotting factors)
Primidone	None known	Hemorrhage
Trimethadione	Mental retardation, facial dysmorphogenesis	Hemorrhage
Cancer Chemotherapy		
Alkylating agents	Abortion, anomalies, CNS effect (?)	Hypoplastic gonads, growth delay, CNS effect (?)
Antimetabolites		
Folic acid analogs (Methotrexate)	Abortion, IUGR, cranial anomalies	Same as above
Pyrimidine analogs (arabinoside)	Same as above	" "
Purine analogs (cytosine, 5-FU)	" "	" "
Antibiotics (actinomycin)	" "	" "
Vinca alkyloids	" "	" "

A.1 (Continued)

Drugs	First Trimester Effects	Second & Third Trimester Effects
Cardiovascular Drugs		
Antihypertensives		
Methyldopa	None known	Hemolytic anemia(?), ileus
Guanethidine	None known	None known
Hydralazine	Skeletal defects(?)	Tachycardia
Propranolol	None known	Bradycardia, hypoglycemia, IUGR with chronic use
Reserpine	None known	Lethargy
Digitalis	None known	Bradycardia
Cold and Cough Preparations		
Antihistamines	None known	None known
Cough suppressants	None known	None known
Decongestants	None known	None known
Expectorants	Fetal goiter (?)	None known
Dextromethorphan	None known	None known
Diuretics		
Furosemide	None known	Death from sudden hypo-perfusion
Thiazides	None known	Thrombocytopenia, hypokalemia, hyperbilirubinemia, hyponatremia, hypovolemia
Fertility Drugs		
Bromocriptine	None known	None known
Clomiphene	Chromosomal abnormalities (?)	Unknown
Hormones		
Androgens	Masculinzation of female fetus	Adrenal suppression (?)
Corticosteroids	Cleft in animals, not in humans	Growth delay
Estrogens	Cardiovascular anomalies	None known
Progestins	Limb reduction; CV anomalies; "VACTERL" Synd.	None known

A.1 (Continued)

Drugs	First Trimester Effects	Second & Third Trimester Effects
Hypoglycemics		
Insulin	Does not cross placenta	None known
Sulfonylureas	Anomalies (?)	Suppressed insulin secretion
Laxatives		
Bisacodyl	None known	None known
Docusate	None known	None known
Mineral oil	Decreased maternal vitamin absorption	Decreased maternal vitamin absorption
Milk of magnesia	None known	None known
Psychoactive Drugs		
Antidepressants (tricyclic)	Limb defects (?)	None known
Benzodiazepines	Oral clefts (?)	Depression, floppy infant
Hydroxyzine	None known	None known
Meprobamate	Cardiac anomalies(?)	None known
Phenothiazines	None known	None known
Sedatives	None known	Depression
Thalidomide	Phocomelia in 20% of cases	None known
Lithium	Facial clefts, Ebstein's anomaly	None known
Thyroid Drugs		
Antithyroid		
^{131}I	Goiter, Abortion, anomalies hypothyroid, mental retardation	Goiter, airway obstruction
Propylthiouracil	Goiter	Same as above
Methimazole	Aplasia cutis, goiter	Same as above, aplasia cutis
Thyroid USP	Does not cross	None known
Thyroxine	Does not cross	None known
Tocolytics		
Alcohol	Fetal alcohol syndrome	Intoxication, hypotonia
Magnesium sulfate	None known	Hypermagnesemia, respiratory depression
Beta agonist sympathomimetics	None known	Tachycardia, hypothermia, hypocalcemia, hypo- and hyperglycemia

A.1 (Continued)

Drugs	First Trimester Effects	Second & Third Trimester Effects
Vaginal Preparations		
Antifungal agents	None known	None known
Podophyllin	Mutagenesis (?)	CNS effects (?)
Vitamins (> RDA?)		
A	Urogenital anomalies (?)	None known
B	None known	None known
C	None known	Scurvy after delivery
D	Mental retardation facial cleft	None known
E	None known	None known
K	None known	None known
Antiasthmatics		
Theophylline	None known	Respiratory distress less likely
Terbutaline	None known	Tachycardia, hypothermia, hypocalcemia, hypo- and hyperglycemia
"Street" Drugs		
LSD	None known	Withdrawal
Marijuana	None known	None known
Methaqualone	None known	Withdrawal
Heroin	None known	Depression, withdrawal
Methadone	None known	Withdrawal
Pentazosine	None known	Withdrawal
Cocaine	None known	Withdrawal
Other		
Cimetidine	None known	None known
Caffeine	Anomalies (?) in high doses	Jitteriness
Azathiaprine	Skeletal defect (?)	None known
Nonoxynol-9	None known	None known
Prostigmin	None known (minimal to cross)	None known
Saccharine	None known	None known
Cis-retinoic acid	Cardiac defects hydrocephalus, ear and hearing defects	None known
Penicillamine	None known	None known

A.2 Drugs in Breast Milk

Drug (Brand)	Neonatal Effect at Maternal Therapeutic Doses

Analgesics and Anti-Inflammatory Drugs

Acetaminophen	Detoxified in liver. Avoid during immediate postpartum period. Otherwise NS.
Aspirin	Transfer to milk not favored. At maternal dose of 12-16 tablets/day, no ill effects on infant. When mother requires high anti-arthritic doses, monitor infant for bruise-ability. May interfere with infant's platelet function.
Codeine	NS
Indomethacin (Indocin)	Used to close patent ductus arteriosus. Insufficient data on the effect on other vessels. May be nephrotoxic.
Meperidine (Demerol)	NS
Propoxyphene (Darvon, Darvocet)	Only symptoms detectable would be failure to feed and drowsiness. If mother taking maximum recommended dosage in a 24 hr period, the infant could receive 1 mg/day, (a significant dose in a neonate).

Antibiotics

Ampicillin	NS. Possibility of allergic sensitization. Can produce candidiasis and diarrhea in infant.
Cefoxitin (Mefoxin)	Infant could receive 0.7 mg/day, NS
Clindamycin (Cleocin)	NS
Erythromycin (Ilosone, E-mycin)	Use not recommended due to its ability to concentrate in milk. Principally excreted in the liver. Infant's liver function is not fully known. Risk of jaundice.

NS = Not significant

A.2 (Continued)

Drug (Brand)	Neonatal Effect at Maternal Therapeutic Doses
Gentamicin (Garamycin)	Not well absorbed from GI tract. May change gut flora. If GI inflammation or diarrhea exists, monitor infant's serum levels to avoid ototoxicity and nephrotoxicity.
Isoniazid	If mother has active tuberculosis, breast-feeding is contraindicated. Monitor signs of isoniazid toxicity.
Metronidazole (Flagyl)	Contraindicated due to possible carcinogenic effect (in animal studies) and high milk concentration.
Nitrofurantoin (Macrodantin)	NS, except in G6PD-deficient infant.
Nystatin (Mycostatin)	None
Penicillin, benzathine Penicillin G, Penicillin VK	NS. Possibility of allergic sensitization.
Sulfisoxazole (Gantrisin)	Same precautions as sulfacetamide. Crosses into breast milk in high concentrations.
Anticoagulants	
Heparin	None
Warfarin (Coumadin)	NS. May safely breastfeed. Monitor PT.
Anticonvulsants	
Carbamazepine (Tegretol)	A 4-kg infant would receive approximately 0.5 mg/kg, which is pharmacologically insignificant.
Ethosuximide	No specific data.
Phenobarbital	Maternal doses of 60-200 mg/day usually safe for infant. May induce hepatic microsomal enzymes; drowsiness in some cases.

NS = Not significant

A.2 (Continued)

Drug (Brand)	Neonatal Effect at Maternal Therapeutic Doses
Magnesium sulfate	Levels in colostrum increase modestly over the first or second day and return to normal by day 3. Calcium levels are unaffected.
Phenytoin (Dilantin)	Usually no effect at maternal doses of 300-600 mg/day. Possibility of enzyme induction. One case report of methemaglobinemia and cyanosis in infant whose mother was taking phenytoin and phenobarbital.
Primidone	Drowsiness and decreased feeding. May cause bleeding due to hypoprothrominemia. Avoid use during lactation.

Antihistamines and Decongestants

Dextropheniramine maleate, with isoephedrine (sustained release tablets) (Drixoral)	One case report of irritability, excessive crying and disturbed sleeping patterns of 5 days duration. Avoid long-acting preparations.
Diphenhydramine (Benadryl)	NS. May cause sedation, decreased feeding, or may produce stimulation and tachycardia.
Pseudoephedrine	NS in usual doses.

Bronchodilators

Theophylline	Usually not significant. Some reports of irritability and insomnia in infant. Premature infants 3-15 days old have an average half-life of 30.2 hr. Caution with sustained drug release theophylline products. Maximum amount of theophylline that an infant could ingest is 8 mg/liter milk per day. Avoid nursing at time of peak maternal serum level.

Cardiovascular Drugs

Digoxin (Lanoxin)	Due to large volume of distribution, the total daily excretion of digoxin in mothers with therapeutic serum concentrations would not exceed 1-2 mcg. This amount is not sufficient to affect the child.

NS = Not significant

A.2 (Continued)

Drug (Brand)	Neonatal Effect at Maternal Therapeutic Doses
Hydralazine (Apresoline)	Jaundice, thrombocytopenia, electrolyte disturbances possible.
Methyldopa (Aldomet)	No specific reports. Excreted in small amounts.
Propranolol (Inderal)	NS at dosages up to 160 mg/day.
Quinidine	Arrhythmias may occur.
Reserpine	May cause nasal stuffiness, lethargy, diarrhea, increased tracheobronchial secretions with difficulty breathing. Also reported to produce galactorrhea.

Diuretics

Chlorothiazide (Diuril)	Risk of dehydration and electrolyte imbalance low. Monitor weight and wet diapers. Occasional urine specific gravity and serum sodium to assure status of infant. May suppress lactation due to dehydration of mother.
Furosemide (Lasix)	None known
Hydrochlorothiazide (Hydrodiuril)	Same precautions as chlorothiazide

Heavy Metals

Iron	Intake of iron is beneficial to mother and infant.

Hormones and Synthetic Substances

Ethinyl estradiol	Not significant if daily dose of 50 mcg or less.
Mestranol	Not significant if daily dose is 50 mcg or less.

NS = Not significant

A.2 (Continued)

Drug (Brand)	Neonatal Effect at Maternal Therapeutic Doses
Progestins (19-nor-testosterone derivatives)	Not significant if maternal daily dose is 2.5 mg or less.
Insulin	Destroyed in infant's GI tract.
Prednisone	Long-term effects unknown. Minimum amount in breast milk. Not likely to cause effect on infant in short course.

Psychotropic Substances

Amitriptyline (Elavil, Endep)	Probably NS, but long half-life and may accumulate. Watch for depression or failure to feed.
Imipramine (Tofranil)	NS at low doses. Unknown at maternal therapeutic blood levels.
Alcohol	Not significant in moderation. Lethargy and prolonged sleeping when mother consumes excessive amounts.
Barbiturates	Usually insufficient, may induce liver microsomal enzymes.
Chlordiazepoxide (Librium)	Amount secreted usually insufficient to affect infant, although CNS depression has been reported.
Diazepam (Valium)	Reports of lethargy and weight loss. Infant most susceptible during first 4 days of life. Hyperbilirubinemia. Most sources do not advise its use during breastfeeding. Drug accumulation may occur.
Caffeine	Accumulates when intake moderate and continual. Causes jitteriness, wakefulness, and irritability.
Dextroamphetamine (Dexedrine)	No effects on infants when given to 103 postpartum women for depression. Avoid long-acting preparations.

NS = Not significant

A.2 (Continued)

Drug (Brand)	Neonatal Effect at Maternal Therapeutic Doses
Flurazepam (Dalmane)	Some sedation, usually not significant.
Marijuana	Conflicting reports; use not recommended. No beneficial effect.
Chlorpromazine (Thorazine)	NS at doses up to 1200 mg/day.
Prochlorperazine (Compazine)	None known
Thioridazine (Mellaril)	None known
Trifluoperazine (Stelazine)	None known
Lithium	NS

Radiopharmaceuticals and Diagnostic Materials

^{131}I	Breast feeding contraindicated after large therapeutic dose, and should be withheld for 24 hr minimum after smaller diagnostic doses. Check milk prior to resuming feeding.
^{131}I-labeled macroaggregated albumin	Discontinue breast feeding for 10-12 days. Extreme avidity for iodine by the thyroid of young infants. 1/10 of the International Commission on Radiological Protection (ICRP) for drinking water reached 10 days after IV dose of 200 mCi.
Iopanoic acid (Telepaque)	No adverse effects. Iodine excretion can cause rash. Probably no problem with a single dose.
Tuberculin test	Tuberculin-sensitive mothers can passively immunize their infants through breast milk. Immunity may last several years.

NS = Not significant

A.2 (Continued)

Drug (Brand)	Neonatal Effect at Maternal Therapeutic Doses

Thyroid Drugs

Methimazole (Tapazole)	Infant could receive 7-16% of maternal dose. Could interfere with thyroid function. Inhibits synthesis of thyroid hormone.
Propylthiouracil	Infant could receive 0.5 mg/day at maternal dose of 600 mg/day. Thought to be harmless. Infant could ingest 0.07% of mother's daily dose.
Levo-thyroxine (Synthroid)	May delay clinical symptoms of congenital hypothyroidism in breast fed infants (neonates). Improves milk supply in hypothyroid mothers. Not contraindicated.

Vaccines

DPT Vaccine	Does not interfere with immunization schedule.
Poliovirus vaccine	Live virus taken orally. Not necessary to withhold nursing. Provide booster after infant no longer nursing.
Rubella virus vaccine	No harm but will not confer passive immunity.
Hepatitis vaccine	No harm

NS = Not significant

Index